LIZ EARLE'S
QUICK GUIDES
Juicing

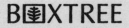

BOXTREE

Acknowledgements

I am grateful to Midi Fairgrieve for helping to produce this book.
I am also indebted to the talented team at Boxtree, Rosemary
Sandberg and Claire Bowles Publicity for their unfailing
enthusiasm and support.

Advice to the Reader

*Before following any dietary advice contained in this book, it is
recommended that you consult your doctor if you suffer from any health
problems or special condition or are in any doubt.*

First published in Great Britain in 1995 by Boxtree Limited,
Broadwall House, 21 Broadwall, London SE1 9PL

The right of Liz Earle to be identified as Author of this Work
has been asserted by her in accordance with the Copyright,
Designs and Patents Act 1988

10 9 8 7 6 5 4 3 2

ISBN: 0 7522 1626 0

Text design by Blackjacks
Cover design by Hammond Hammond

Printed and bound in Great Britain by
Caledonian International Book Manufacturing Ltd, Glasgow

A CIP catalogue entry for this book is available from
the British Library

Contents

Introduction

It would be easy to dismiss juicing as yet another modern health fad, but there is much more to it than that. Juicing is a wonderful way to improve our energy levels, restore vitality and give our bodies a boost. Just how far you take the principle of juicing is up to you. A glass of freshly squeezed orange juice may be all you can manage – or, alternatively, you may find yourself hooked on the idea, investing in a centrifugal juice extractor and juicing everything from alfalfa sprouts to wheatgrass. Juicing is fun, fast and perfect for every member of the family, from baby's first few sips of pressed apples to grandma's antioxidant tonic. Whatever your own needs, I hope you find this *Quick Guide* an invaluable source of juicing inspiration.

Liz Earle

— 1 —
Why Juice?

Fresh juices have the power to nourish, cleanse, protect, soothe and heal. They are nutritious and easy to digest and give us life energy in a naturally delicious drink. It makes sense then to drink fresh juices every day.

There has always been much debate about the relationship between healthy eating and freedom from disease. Some people think there is little or no relationship between the two; while various naturopaths and dietary experts believe our nutritional well-being is the pivot upon which health and disease balance. We do know that many of the chronic diseases common among people on typical 'Western' diets, such as colon cancer, high blood pressure and diabetes, are almost unheard of among certain other cultures with different eating habits. It is thought that a diet high in refined sugars and starches is largely responsible for such diseases.

Modern food is getting less and less healthy as we demand greater returns from crops and more refined and processed 'convenience foods'. Commercial farming is intensive and competitive and uses chemical fertilisers and pesticides to sustain high yields. This not only robs the soil of nutrients, but leaves harmful chemical residues in the growing plants. Food processing further depletes and destroys vital nutrients, so by the time food gets to our table there is not much of the original goodness left. Juicing can make the essential difference between being under-nourished or well-nourished.

Although there is much research still to be done in the area of nutrition and health, many health experts and practitioners believe that nutritional deficiencies are one of the most common contributors to disease in our time. So many people in the developed world are not following a healthy life plan of wholesome, balanced eating and regular exercise that it is not surprising we suffer from a long list of chronic complaints, ranging from arthritis and diabetes to coronary heart disease and cancer.

Health isn't something that can be turned on or off overnight. It is not what we eat or drink occasionally that determines our well-being, but what we consume every day. That is why it is so important to eat natural, well-balanced foods, fresh from nature's garden. Fresh fruit and vegetable juices form a valuable part of any dietary journey back to health and happiness and their greatest benefit is derived when combined with a healthy diet, positive thinking, correct breathing and regular exercise.

Really, the drinking of fresh juices is a wonderfully healthy habit. It is because juices are so easily digested and assimilated that they have such a health-building impact on the body. We can make maximum use of the nutrients with minimum expense to the digestive system. Juices have the power to protect us from illness by strengthening the immune system. They cleanse the blood and vital organs and stimulate our metabolism. All these things help to maintain a healthy, vibrant body.

Why not buy fresh juices?

The simple answer is that many of them are not what they appear to be! For example, in 1987 an American juice company pleaded guilty to charges of selling millions of bottles of artificially flavoured water labelled as 100 percent pure apple juice!

Other juice manufacturers import cheap fruit from countries which are still using banned pesticides like DDT. Minute traces of these chemicals penetrate the growing fruit and eventually end up in our bodies!

To get the most value out of fresh juices they really need to be consumed within a couple of hours, otherwise they lose vitality and nutrients. Within twenty-four hours, for example, a glass of carrot juice can lose as much as half of its vitamins, minerals and trace elements. Leaving a juice to stand means that the enzyme activity is also vastly reduced. Enzymes are the things which help chemical reactions take place in the body, which means they are vital to proper digestion. How many shop-bought juices are less than a few hours old? Most are pasteurised or sterilised to give them a longer shelf life. These processes involve high temperatures, which not only destroy the active enzymes but some of the nutrients as well, effectively rendering it 'dead food'.

Other ready-made juices contain a host of additives from colourings and flavourings to corn syrup, salt and chemical preservatives.

Having said all that, some ready-made juices are fine – it is a case of being discerning, armed with the knowledge that 'fresh is best'.

Eleven Good Reasons to Juice

* Juices can help to keep us beautiful.
* Juices are rich in active enzymes which aid digestion.
* Juices are packed with essential vitamins and minerals.
* Juices boost our vitality.
* Juices help to eliminate toxins.
* Juices are rich in antioxidants which protect from disease and premature ageing.
* Juices contain essential amino acids.
* Juices are rich in chlorophyll.
* Juices help balance the body's acid/alkaline levels.
* Juices help in weight reduction.
* Fresh juice tastes great!

THE BEAUTY FACTOR

Beauty, like health, comes from within, and so what we eat plays a vital role here. There is only so much we can do on the outside to stay looking good, but nothing will last if it doesn't come from within. Sparkling eyes, lovely skin, vim and vigour are all signs of a healthy working system. Raw fruit and vegetable juices aid the body's natural functions of cleansing and repair which keep us looking young and feeling great.

It's really not surprising that juices are so popular when you stop to consider how well they can help us to achieve optimum health and vitality and keep us looking young and beautiful!

RICH IN ACTIVE ENZYMES

Without enzymes we cannot digest our food properly and this factor alone makes them vital to health.

Enzymes are catalysts, which means they assist in chemical reactions. You could think of them as a highly efficient labour force which is constantly breaking down and rebuilding bits of the body. At any one time, millions of them are working together metabolising our food and renewing our cells.

Without enzymes, the human body would be lifeless. A lack of enzymes means that we cannot convert our food into energy or transform carbohydrates, proteins, fats, vitamins and minerals into muscle, bone, hair, organs, skin and so on. Enzyme deficiency leads to a situation where we are literally starving in the midst of plenty because we cannot get what we need from our food.

When our natural enzyme level gets too low, our metabolism slows, we get tired and all our bodily functions begin to suffer. Cells are not repaired and renewed efficiently which means we age more quickly. The more we can conserve our own natural enzymes by eating food which is raw and alive, the healthier we will be and the longer we will live. It is only by eating raw food that we can replenish and preserve our own enzymes.

When you consider what is actually involved in digesting food from beginning to end you can appreciate how much energy it takes. That's why people often feel tired after a large meal as their body is using most of its energy for digestion. It is vitally important to consume enough live enzymes in the form of raw foods to leave plenty of energy for other bodily functions such as fighting disease and detoxification. If we use up all the body's available energy for digestion we cannot eliminate toxins properly which leads to a range of health problems from cellulite to cancer.

This is one of the reasons why many health and beauty experts advocate fresh juice fasts as a way of conserving the body's energy for use in cleansing and renewal.

Many enzymes rely in some way on other nutrients to be present, such as vitamins and minerals, before a chemical reaction can take place. These nutrients are known as co-factors. Raw food provides us with the complete package of enzymes and co-factors needed to break down that particular food and release its valuable nutrients and vitality.

Enzymes are sensitive to heat and are destroyed by high temperatures. They can also be damaged by exposure to air and by freezing.

Essentially, many of us eat dead food because the active component has been destroyed. Freshly squeezed juices give us live enzymes, complete with their co-factors. The more enzymes we consume the better nourished our cells will be, so we can live a healthier, happier and longer life.

PACKED WITH ESSENTIAL VITAMINS

Like enzymes, vitamins are essential to life; therefore, if you are completely deficient of one or more vitamins, you will die. Don't panic though – in most cases vitamin deficiencies are easy to spot. Vitamins are widely available in food and if we eat a well-balanced diet we are sure to get adequate supplies.

Generally, vitamins fall into two groups – the water-soluble vitamins which include the B vitamins and vitamin C, and the fat-soluble vitamins which include vitamins A, D, E and K. The body can store the fat-soluble vitamins for a limited amount of time, but the water-soluble ones need to be constantly replenished.

Vitamin deficiency

Because vitamins are essential for life they have an amazing impact on our health. Without adequate supplies, enzyme efficiency is decreased, and we can fall prey to a host of vitamin-deficiency diseases like beriberi, scurvy and reproductive abnormalities.

A deficiency of the water-soluble vitamins is more likely than of the fat-soluble vitamins because the former are generally not stored in the body for long periods of time (apart from vitamin B12).

Who is at risk from deficiency?

Individual vitamin requirements vary from person to person and with each stage of life. For most people the recommended daily allowances (see below) are a reasonably good guide to how much you need; however, some people will need more than this, for example pregnant or breastfeeding women, the elderly, infants and young children, and people with particular lifestyles and diets such as vegetarians and vegans, smokers and alcoholics.

Many other factors affect our vitamin status including an inadequate diet, impaired digestion, overcooking, canning, processing, bad storage of food and irradiation. Added to these are poor diet and lifestyle factors which can further rob the body of these valuable nutrients.

Fresh juices provide one of the best ways of consuming adequate supplies of vitamins with the minimum of loss or destruction. They provide them in a balanced form together with their mineral co-factors.

How much do we need?

There are generally agreed Recommended Daily Allowances for the important vitamins and minerals – known as RDAs. However, many nutritionists feel that these RDA figures represent, at best, a *minimum* daily allowance because commercially grown foods have, in most cases, lost substantial nutrient value. The twice Nobel Prize winning nutrition scientist, Dr Linus Pauling, states that 'Doctors claim that the ordinary diet will give you all the vitamins you need – this is not true – we do not get the amounts needed in the average diet, which does not contain all the nutrients we need for good health.' The author Beata Bishop, who successfully won her battle against cancer by following the Gerson Therapy diet, also believes the average Western diet to be inadequate, and says that 'not only is our appearance at stake, but the fundamentals of good health are at risk'.

In order to stay healthy you really need to make sure that you get *at least* the RDA of the important minerals and vitamins, and juices can help you to do this. Table 1.1 shows the RDAs and uses of the essential vitamins, with good food sources.

PACKED WITH ESSENTIAL MINERALS

Like vitamins, minerals are essential to good health and many of us are familiar with the relationship between zinc and a healthy skin and that of iron and healthy blood.

Minerals can also be split into two groups – the major minerals, and the minor or trace minerals. The major minerals include calcium, magnesium, sodium, potassium, phosphorus, sulphur and chlorine. We also need others, in smaller amounts, and these are known as minor or trace minerals. They include

TABLE 1.1 VITAMINS

Vitamin & RDA	Needed for	Good sources
Fat soluble A 2,500iu	Growth; healthy skin, lungs, eyes and eyesight; helps in fighting infection.	Yellow/orange/red/dark green fruit and vegetables.
E 15iu	Aids reproduction; protects against heart disease; acts as an antioxidant.	Cabbage, Brussels sprouts, green leafy vegetables, sprouted seeds and beans.
K 300–500mcg	Blood clotting.	Green leafy vegetables.
Water soluble B complex (there are many B vitamins)	Healthy nervous system; carbohydrate, protein and fat metabolism; healthy hair, skin and eyes; red blood-cell formation; aids proper liver function.	Dark green vegetables, citrus fruit, strawberries.
Bioflavonoids (no known RDA)	Help to increase strength of capillaries.	Citrus fruits, blackcurrants.
C 45mg	Immune system; wound healing; fighting infection; healthy bones and teeth; guards against stress; an antioxidant.	Citrus fruits, broccoli, potatoes, green peppers, tomatoes.
Folic acid 400mcg	Red blood-cell formation; protein metabolism; foetal growth; nervous system.	Dark green leafy vegetables.

iu – International Units; mg – milligrams; mcg – micrograms zinc, iron, chromium, copper, fluorine, silicon, iodine, manganese, selenium, nickel, tin, vanadium, molybdenum, cobalt – and even arsenic!

It's this complex of major and minor minerals that bestows the quality to our food and there is no greater natural source than fresh fruit and vegetables.

Deficiency

Most vitamin deficiencies can be corrected fairly quickly; this isn't true for minerals though. We can build up long-term deficiencies where the effects are gradual and insidious. A chromium deficiency, for example, may show up eventually as bouts of fatigue, exhaustion and hunger. Magnesium deficiency can lead to premenstrual tension (PMT), depression, muscle tremors and disorientation. Zinc deficiency can lead to infertility. Iron deficiency is one of the most prevalent mineral deficiencies and affects one-fifth of the world's population. It is very common in women who lose iron with their monthly period. Symptoms include anaemia, brittle nails, weakness, fatigue and breathing impairment. Vegetarian and vegan diets often lack enough iron in the diet since meat is most people's main source.

Correcting mineral deficiencies takes much longer than correcting vitamin deficiencies, so it is essential that we always meet our daily requirements. Juices can help you to do this, while at the same time improving your skin, hair, nails and moods! Table 1.2 shows the RDAs and uses of the essential minerals, together with good food sources.

HIGH IN VITALITY

When was the last time you felt really vibrant? Ready to run a mile or climb a mountain? That long?

In order to have high vitality we need to eat high-vitality foods. This means eating foods that are alive and packed with active enzymes, vitamins, minerals and other essential nutrients.

Many of us may have forgotten what true vitality feels like as we get more and more used to a diet and lifestyle which encourages a lack of energy.

How do juices rate?

On a vitality scale of one to ten, raw foods and juices come at the top, while processed and tinned foods sit at the bottom. As a naturopathic rule of thumb, the fresher the food, the more vitality it contains.

Juices are great energy boosters. They are rapidly digested in the stomach and taken up by the blood. This makes their journey round the body, nourishing and revitalising the cells, a speedy and efficient process.

Harbouring vitality for healing

Dr Max Gerson, MD, who founded the Gerson Institute for cancer treatment, found that his patients tended to recover from degenerative illness when put on a diet made up largely of fresh raw juices. After years of dietary experimentations, he designed the stringent Gerson Therapy programme which includes ten fresh juices per day.

Apart from measurable things like vitamins, minerals, flavours and so on, plants also contain something that is not easily measured which aids in the healing process. It is this intangible or subtle energy that provides the life spark in all living organisms. The more raw food we eat, the more of this life energy we receive.

This is why raw fruit and vegetable juice can help you rediscover the energy you once had and the health you thought you had lost, as well as giving you the radiant glow of a healthy functioning body. Vibrant health makes us feel literally intoxicated with life and gives us the drive to fulfil our goals.

TABLE 1.2 MINERALS

Vitamin & RDA	Needed for	Good sources
Calcium 800mg	Strong, healthy bones and teeth; muscle action; nerve function; normal blood clotting.	Dark green leaves, especially kale and turnip tops.
Iodine 150mcg	Production of thyroxine which regulates metabolism and energy production, needed for physical and mental development.	Green leafy vegetables, cabbage, pineapple.
Iron 8–10mg	Healthy blood, haemoglobin production, oxygenating the blood; promotes growth.	Green vegetables, beetroot, apricots, prunes.
Magnesium 350–450mg	Healthy bones and muscles (works with calcium); blood sugar control.	Dark green vegetables.
Phosphorus 800mg	Builds and maintains bones and teeth, nervous tissue and hair; helps with absorption of fats and carbohydrates.	Asparagus, carrots, endive, kale, parsnips, potatoes, spinach, watercress.
Potassium 2–6g	Muscle contraction; nerve transmission; healthy skin; water balance (works with sodium).	Most vegetables and fruit.
Selenium 150mcg	Antioxidant.	Broccoli, tomatoes.
Sodium 1.5g	Muscle contraction; nerve transmission; fluid balance.	Carrots, endive, parsley.

g – grams; mg – milligrams; mcg – micrograms

ELIMINATION OF TOXINS

It is the cleansing ability of fresh fruit and vegetable juices that makes them a must for all detoxification diets. Some are more aggressive in their cleansing action than others, but as a rough guide, juices from vegetables and sprouted seeds and beans are mild cleansers, whereas fruit juices are strong cleansers.

How do juices work?

Juices have the ability to scour away waste and harmful bacteria from the cells which means they can cleanse at a very deep level. It is the various fruit acids that do most of the cleansing. For example, tartaric acid, found abundantly in grapes and pineapples, inhibits the growth of some harmful moulds and bacteria. While malic acid, found in apples, apricots, lemons, peaches, prunes, plums and other fruits, is an excellent natural antiseptic, and helps to cleanse the intestines, kidneys, liver and stomach. Citric acid is probably the best-known fruit acid, found in the highest quantities in citrus fruits, and is one of the strongest acid cleansers.

It is because juices are such efficient cleansers that they have been used by naturopaths for many years to help cleanse and restore sick bodies back to health. As part of a daily regime, fresh juices can help to keep your system working efficiently and free from waste, making it much harder for unwelcome things like cellulite to take a hold. (See Chapter 6 for further details on juice fasting and detox diets.)

AMINO ACIDS

Fresh fruit and vegetables enrich the diet with amino acids in an easily digestible form. Amino acids are the building blocks of protein. They work hand in hand with enzymes and are responsible for an array of diverse functions, from the making of hormones to building muscle, blood and organs. One of their key functions is the digestion and assimilation of food, and if this doesn't happen, other bodily functions begin to suffer. A deficiency of amino acids can cause a range of symptoms from digestive disorders and allergies to premature ageing.

Raw fruit and vegetable juices help to bridge the gap between health and illness by supplying a daily dose of essential amino acids. Juices made from leafy greens and sprouts are especially rich in amino acids.

CHLOROPHYLL

We find chlorophyll in abundance in all green plants. It's the stuff which enables plants to turn sunlight into food and without it they wouldn't be able to grow. It stands at the base of all food chains.

Because chlorophyll is able to trap the sun's energy and use it for growth, this same energy gets transmitted, through the food chain, to every living creature on the planet – and that includes us!

What can it do for us?

Chlorophyll provides us with life energy. It cleans the system, builds the blood and cells and makes a wonderful all-round regenerative tonic. (How many of us could survive without the occasional one of these?) One of the best ways to get high amounts of chlorophyll into the diet is by drinking green juices, in particular alfalfa, wheatgrass, leafy greens, watercress, green peppers, celery and cucumbers. Not surprisingly, four green juices per day are included in the Gerson Cancer Therapy diet.

BALANCING ALKALINES AND ACIDS

Fruit and vegetable juices help us maintain and restore the correct acid/alkaline balance in the body. In a strange paradox, acid foods have an alkalinising effect on the body, while alkaline foods have an acid effect on the body. Therefore, if we eat acidic foods, the ultimate effect on the body is alkalinising!

Why is this important?
High acidity is what we get with chronic complaints and many of us eat too much acid-forming food such as meat and dairy products. These foods unbalance the body's natural acid/alkaline balance which leads to all sorts of health problems. Western diets are particularly acid forming; added to which, lifestyle factors such as stress and overwork further increase the acid load. A typical Western diet, high in animal proteins, refined sugar and flour, chemical additives and drugs, causes acids to build up in the cells eventually leading to complaints such as arthritis or gout. Acid cells attract toxins which in turn make the cells more acidic. One of the main causes of fatigue is acidity of the blood and it's well known that cancer cells enjoy an acid environment.

What can we do?
You've guessed it – eat more fruit and vegetables! In this respect juices really come into their own and provide a delicious way to keep the balance right. In general fruit, especially citrus, comes out top in its alkalinising effects on the body.

RICH IN ANTIOXIDANTS
Antioxidants are the things that have been hailed as the secret to living longer and looking younger. The three main antioxidant nutrients are vitamin A (or more accurately its vegetable precursor beta-carotene), vitamin C and vitamin E. Each has a protective effect on the other, which basically means that their combined power is greater than the same amount of any of them singly.

In terms of health, there is much medical evidence to show that antioxidants can help to prevent cancer, cardiovascular disease and other chronic diseases. There have been literally hundreds of studies into the extraordinary powers of beta-carotene, vitamin C and vitamin E with impressive results. For example, a study carried out in Finland over a twenty-five-year period on 4,500 men concluded that those with the highest intake of these three antioxidants had the lowest level of lung cancer. Even among the non-smokers, it was found that those taking the lowest levels of these three vitamins were at least twice as likely to develop lung cancer as those receiving the highest levels of the vitamins.

Another study of 500 men in Scotland found that the higher the levels of beta-carotene, vitamin C and vitamin E in their bloodstream, the lower the risk of angina. This study concluded that 'populations with a high incidence of coronary heart disease may benefit from eating diets rich in natural antioxidants, particularly vitamin E'.

How do they work?

Antioxidants do the job of mopping up the baddies in the body, called free radicals. Free radicals are formed as a result of normal bodily function, but an excess causes problems. To understand why they are so damaging, we need to understand how they work. Basically, free radicals are highly unstable substances which react with and damage other molecules. It is these damaged molecules that have been linked to almost every degenerative disease, from cell destruction and tumour growth to enzyme damage. In fact, research in this area suggests that free radicals are a major contributor towards at least fifty of our most prevalent diseases including heart and lung disease, certain cancers, cataracts, rheumatoid arthritis, even the ageing process itself.

We can see the damaging effects of free radicals in action by watching a freshly sliced apple turn brown. This happens when the exposed apple comes into contact with the air and begins to oxidise. However, if you squeeze some lemon juice on the apple it protects it from damage because the vitamin C in the lemon juice acts as an antioxidant.

How can we protect ourselves?
Antioxidants are the key to protection against free-radical damage. They travel round the body scavenging and mopping up excess free radicals. We can use them in the war against these nasties while at the same time avoiding factors which encourage the formation of free radicals, such as pollution, smoking, barbecued foods, fried foods, ultraviolet radiation and alcohol.

Fresh fruit and vegetable juices are an excellent way of making sure we get enough antioxidants in our daily diet to fight against free-radical damage inside the body. All fresh fruit and vegetable juices are an excellent source of these wonderful vitamins. The Gerson Cancer Therapy diet includes ten fresh fruit and vegetable juices every day in the fight against disease.

Vitamin A as an antioxidant
There are two types of vitamin A – retinol, which is generally found in animal foods, especially organ meats like liver – and beta-carotene, found in fruit and vegetables. High doses of retinol can be toxic, whereas beta-carotene is perfectly safe. Beta-carotene can be converted easily by the body into retinol and therefore adequate supplies of beta-carotene provide plenty of retinol. The excess is used as an antioxidant. Vitamin A's ability to act as a free-radical scavenger is strongest in the lining of the tissues and has been shown to prevent cancer formation. This vitamin is also vital in protecting the thymus gland which is one of the immune system's most important organs. Beta-carotene is found in all fruit and vegetables and is especially high in yellow and orange fruit and vegetables and dark green leaves.

Vitamin C as an antioxidant
Citrus fruits, potatoes, green leaves and tomatoes are great sources of vitamin C and it is one of the most protective substances we have. It strengthens the immune system and helps to fight infections and heal wounds.

Vitamin E as an antioxidant

Vitamin E works best against damaged fats and is particularly effective in reducing wrinkled tissues and damaged cells from smoking tobacco. Rich sources of vitamin E are found in fresh beets, celery and green vegetables, especially watercress.

There are other nutrients which complete the antioxidant 'team', namely the trace mineral selenium, and the amino acid cysteine, both of which are found in fruit and vegetables. Broccoli and tomatoes are high in selenium, whereas cysteine is plentiful in beetroot, carrots, cabbage, kale, apple, pineapple and raspberries.

Selenium works well with vitamin E which is why these two are often hailed as the anti-ageing nutrients. Selenium's protective functions have also been found to lessen the risk of heart disease and cancer and both these conditions are found to be much higher in areas of the world with low levels of selenium in the soil.

HELP IN WEIGHT REDUCTION

Juices are virtually fat free, low in calories and packed with vital nutrients which makes them a valuable addition to any weight-loss regime. They also help to curb the appetite and speed up the metabolism.

And they taste great too!

—2—

Getting Started

Now that you know *why* fresh juices are such an enriching feature of the diet, it's time to get started. A well-thought-out juicing programme can be the first step towards a new you!

Equipment

The first thing you need to do, if you don't already have one, is buy a juicer, and if you are planning to venture beyond citrus juice you will need one of the high-speed electric juicers. These not only work for citrus fruits but can also extract juice from hard fruit and vegetables such as carrots, beetroot, apples and potatoes.

It is always a good idea to check with the supplier whether the juicer can be washed in a dishwasher, since high temperatures can warp some plastic parts.

There are several good quality juicers on the market,* the most popular being the **centrifugal juicers** which have revolutionised juice making. These have an electrically driven high-speed blade which separates the juice from the pulp. The juice goes into one container and the pulp into another. Centrifugal juicers are also relatively inexpensive and easy to clean, which makes them an attractive choice for any kitchen.

The four most popular centrifugal machines at the time of writing are the Moulinex Compact Juice Extractor, the Moulinex Juice Extractor, the Braun Compact Juice Extractor

---

* All prices are correct at the time of going to press. See Useful Addresses for stockists.

and the Kenwood Centrifuge. They can be found in most department stores and cost between £35 and £40. All of these claim to be easy to clean and have an automatic separation of juice and pulp. At the more expensive end of the centrifugal juicer market is the Vita-mine Centrifugal Juicer, at around £130, which can extract proportionally more juice than the less expensive models because it has a much more powerful motor. Or there is the Maynard Professional Juicer at around £199.

Top of the range are the more expensive **masticating juicers** which mash the fruit and vegetables before squeezing the juice through a stainless steel sieve. They are much more efficient than centrifugal juicers and can extract up to 25 percent more juice. It's worth noting here that the more juice that is extracted from a single piece of fruit or vegetable, the higher its concentration of nutrients. This is why those following the Gerson Cancer Therapy diet need to use a high-quality masticating juicer to get maximum health benefits (such as the Champion Juicer, which costs around £350).

If you are intending to go the whole hog and juice from wheatgrass, herbs and sprouted beans and seeds as well, then you may want to consider buying a juicer such as the Health Fountain Juicer. This type of machine is better suited to extracting juice from stringy, fibrous material like wheatgrass, hailed for its high chlorophyll content, or herbs such as parsley, which is rich in iron and vitamin C. The Health Fountain Juicer costs around £120. This machine will also juice apples and carrots, etc., but it is more time consuming to use than the Champion or Vita-mine.

As the name implies, a **citrus press** is only for citrus fruit, and so it has obvious limitations for a juicing revolution in your home. The three most commonly sold at the time of writing are the Krups Citrus Press, the Moulinex Citrus Press and the Braun Citrus Press. These all cost between £15 and £18 and are available in most department stores.

Fruit and Vegetables

The other thing to do is to establish a good source of fresh fruit and vegetables, so it's worth having a scout around your local area to see what is available.

To get the best out of fruit and vegetables they should be organic. Organically grown crops are free from harmful fertilisers and pesticides and contain a natural balance of the complete range of soil nutrients which commercial farming depletes. For example, artificial fertilisers can cause elements such as calcium and magnesium to be so diluted in the soil that they are not taken up by the plants. Pesticides can affect our digestion and interfere with the absorption of nutrients from food. Although all pesticides are tested by MAFF (Ministry of Agriculture, Food and Fisheries), many of those used today were approved when standards were comparatively lax and we still don't know what are the long-term effects of low doses or of cocktails of these chemicals.

FACTS ABOUT PESTICIDES:

* 600 pesticides are permitted in the European Union.
* 98 percent of British vegetables and cereals are sprayed with pesticides.
* In 1982 one English lettuce crop was sprayed forty-eight times with four different pesticides.
* In 1992 the MAFF Monitoring Service discovered that one-third of British carrots contained the pesticide Triazophos above the maximum residue level.
* Pesticide residues have been found in human breast milk.

FACTS ABOUT ORGANICALLY GROWN FOOD:

* Contains higher levels of vitamins, minerals and nutrients.
* Free of traces of chemical fertilisers and pesticides.
* Tastes better.
* Better for the environment.

If you have trouble finding an organic source, then the Soil Association can provide a list of organic farmers and suppliers in your area (see Useful Addresses). There are quite a few consumer cooperatives and box-delivery schemes around, so it is worth checking to see if there is one near you.

However, it is not always possible to get hold of organic produce, and the next best thing is to buy locally grown produce. At least this way, if you can't avoid possible residues of synthetic chemicals, you can ensure that the nutrient content hasn't been depleted by early harvesting or lengthy storage. The longer a fruit or vegetable is transported or stored, the faster it deteriorates.

Produce from abroad is often picked well before it ripens which means it has less time to gather essential nutrients from the soil. By buying locally grown fruit and vegetables in season it helps us to keep in touch with the ebb and flow of nature's cycle and ensure we get the nutrients we need when we need them. Don't be afraid to ask your local supplier or supermarket where their produce comes from. Local greengrocers normally have a good idea of where their fruit and vegetables are grown and they might even be persuaded to stock organic produce.

Ideally, grow your own for the ultimate in fresh, tasty juices.

REMEMBER:

* The fresher the fruit and vegetables, the richer they are in nutrients.
* The freer they are of harmful chemicals, the more nutritious they are likely to be.

SHOPPING TIPS:

* Buy organic produce if possible or buy local produce that is in season.
* Shop frequently to ensure fresh and ripe produce.
* Throw away mouldy, bruised or overripe produce.
* Don't buy irradiated produce.
* Keep fruit and vegetables stored in a cool, dry place.

—— 3 ——
Juice Therapy

Food has been used to heal the sick for centuries and many people will be familiar with the saying of Hippocrates, father of medicine, 'Let food be your medicine, and your medicine be your food.' Apples and prunes make excellent laxatives, cabbage juice helps to soothe and cure peptic ulcers, and watermelons and cucumbers are wonderful natural diuretics. It is this potential for juices to be therapeutic as well as nutritious that has led many naturopaths to use them as curative therapy.

To a great extent we are what we eat. The food we put into our body determines the health of every single cell. It is so important then to eat food that is fresh and alive in order to build healthy tissues and organs and to keep the body working properly. Consuming raw, natural, uncooked food is the key to building and maintaining health, which is why fresh juices are one of the best ways to keep well. If we feed our bodies with the maximum amount of nutrients and the minimum of toxins, we can ensure a long and healthy life.

Fruits are revitalisers and cleansers and help to keep the channels of elimination functioning properly, while vegetables are the building blocks of life and are cleansing and restorative. This is why raw fruit and vegetables have been used by naturopaths for so long, since they underpin the nature cure principles of cleansing and restoration in an effort to stimulate self-healing.

The European naturopath, Dr Bircher-Benner, who founded the famous Bircher-Benner Clinic, said that 'nothing more therapeutic exists on Earth than green juices'. Both Dr

Bircher-Benner and Dr Max Gerson have devised treatment programmes which use large quantities of fresh juice.

Nature's curative powers are concentrated in fresh fruit and vegetable juices, which is why they are used to restore the sick to health and to keep the healthy from getting sick.

Fasting

Fasting is one of the oldest forms of natural health cure and references to fasting can be found in the Bible and other religious tomes. Not only does absence from food give a boost to the physical body, but it also helps to cleanse and renew the spirit. Many religious fasts were, and still are, undertaken for this reason – to help devotees reach new spiritual awareness and overcome the desires of the flesh. Dr Otto Buchinger, who developed the Buchinger method of fasting, said, 'The world of prayer, in fact religions generally, and the world of fasting are closely related. Indeed, each one promotes the other.' Fasting is certainly an all-embracing treatment affecting body and soul at the same time.

The principles of fasting are very simple – restoration of the body through cleansing. This is why fasting is so often advocated by nature cure practitioners in order to stimulate the process of self-healing. We do have the ability to detoxify our systems, but in today's world we are bombarded with toxins – from environmental pollutants and agricultural chemicals to rancid fats and food additives. If these poisons are not eliminated, they circulate around the body and overload the liver, kidneys, lungs, skin and colon. Others lodge themselves within cells and tissues and eventually cause disease. Fasting helps to remove these long-stored toxins and return the body to health. It is one of the most ancient forms of healing and traditionally has been used to cure a wide range of illnesses such as asthma, bronchitis, rheumatism, obesity, migraines, acne, liver problems, constipation, gallstones and tumours.

Without obstacles in its way like using excessive energy in digesting and processing food, the body will self-heal and eliminate poisons and rebalance its internal chemistry. We have a vital force within us that can heal as long as that vitality is not being exhausted by an overburdened digestive and eliminative system, pollution, stress and bad living. Fasting gives the body a chance to wake up its latent curative powers and rejuvenate body, mind and spirit.

Fasting forms one of the mainstays of naturopathic principles and is widely used in natural health care. Dr Zabel, a fasting specialist, stated that 'Hardly any other healing method reaches so deeply into a sick body as fasting.' Dr Max Gerson brought the ancient principles of fasting back into popular use as a powerful form of treatment against cancer when he developed the Gerson Therapy based on raw food and juices. Inspired by the work of Max Gerson, the American 'Juiceman', Jay Korvich, cured himself of a serious illness by drinking thirteen glasses of carrot and apple juice every day for two and a half years. That was forty years ago, and since then he has dedicated his life to spreading the word about the wonders of juicing. He believes that fasting cleanses the body and refreshes the soul.

Fasting can be used both as a treatment of chronic diseases, and as a preventative therapy. It is of course far better to prevent illness, than to find a cure for it.

When animals get sick or ill, they fast until they begin to feel better again. We can learn a lot from this basic instinct. Quite simply, fasting gives the body a rest from the never-ending cycle of digestion, assimilation and elimination. It gives the body some breathing space in which to flush out the back-log of toxins. During a fast the body is able to cleanse, purify and rebuild itself. Longer fasts, of more than a few days, can result in deep cleansing at tissue level where accumulated toxins and wastes have built up over long periods of time. If the body is constantly dealing with the daily process of digestion, assimilation and elimination, it doesn't have the spare energy to remove toxins at this deeper level.

Fasting is a day off from the normal bodily processes, in which the body can cleanse, purify and resurrect itself – and we all need the occasional day off. During a fast the system is able to flush out the liver, kidneys and bladder and generally purge the system. Fasting is both appealing and challenging and can be a time for looking inward and assessing possible life changes. It gives you time to assess where you are and what you want to achieve. In a nutshell, fasting offers the chance to cleanse the inner person and the outer person.

WHO CAN FAST?

Fasting is largely harmless and anyone who wants better health and greater energy can have a go. People with chronic conditions like diabetes, heart disease, liver disease, cancer, the elderly and pregnant women should always consult their doctor before undertaking a fast, even a one-day fast. However, most healthy people can safely fast for between one and three days, but if you have any worries at all then have a word with your doctor or an experienced practitioner before starting.

Fasting is a great preventative measure and can make the difference between health and disease. Just like any other regular cleaning process, from spring cleaning our homes to washing our clothes, the body needs to be cleaned too. Fasting increases energy and extends our life expectancy – in fact, in a study carried out on mice who were regularly fasted, the results showed that their lifespan was increased by 40 percent.

JUICE FASTING

Strictly speaking, a fast is the complete absence of food, but water may be drunk freely. Juices have the advantage over water in that not only do they flush out the system, they also nurture and strengthen the body with vitality and nutrients.

Short juice fasts of up to three days are a wonderful way to rid the body of toxins and boost the eliminative system. Juice fasts stimulate the whole metabolic process which means that excess weight falls off, your skin becomes clearer, your hair shines, eyes brighten and the intestines and other essential organs purge themselves of waste.

By drinking fresh juices you are already bypassing part of the digestive process which separates liquid from bulk, and this makes digestion less taxing on the body as a whole. At the same time your body receives the maximum amount of life-giving enzymes and nutrients in just a few minutes. An abundance of live, uncooked foods flushes toxins out of the body and leaves you feeling refreshed and energised. Freshly made juices contain about 95 percent of the food value of whole fruit and vegetables and this package of nutrients, enzymes and vitality is instantly released into the body through the bloodstream. The road to health and vitality begins with cleansing and regenerating your whole body, and juice fasting can form a first step in that process (see Chapter 6).

—— 4 ——
A–Z of Juicing

This chapter describes forty of the most commonly juiced fruits and vegetables, with a guide to their health and healing powers. Vegetables are listed alphabetically, followed by fruits. Generally speaking, fruits are considered to be a better source of vitamins than vegetables, while vegetables are considered to be a better source of minerals than fruits. (Refer to the nutrient composition table for details of the individual fruits and vegetables listed in this A–Z.) Fruits are highly eliminative, especially citrus fruits, pineapples and grapes; vegetables have a milder cleansing action on the body and are extremely restorative.

Vegetables

ASPARAGUS
Asparagus is a member of the lily family which includes other vegetables like onions, leeks and garlic. It was popular in Roman times and was thought to have strong aphrodisiac powers! Whether that is the case or not, asparagus is a good source of folic acid and vitamin E, both of which are strongly associated with sexual drive and performance. Asparagus is a highly alkaline food and so is considered a good vegetable in elimination diets. It cleanses the blood and tissues of waste and helps to dissolve kidney stones. According to juice authority Norman Walker DSc, asparagus juice helps to break up oxalic acid crystals in the kidneys and muscles which makes it useful in treating rheumatism. Green-tipped asparagus is high in vitamin

A which improves hair, skin and eyes, and guards against cancer. Many of the elements which have a beneficial building effect on the liver, kidneys, skin and bones are found in asparagus, including vitamins A, B1, C, E, choline, folic acid and potassium. Raw juice makes a particularly effective diuretic and mixes well with carrot and cucumber in this respect.

Buying and preparing: Look for bright green asparagus with firm, fresh tips. Do not buy stalks that are old and woody or limp looking. The UK asparagus season is from about April to early July. Asparagus will keep for a few days in the fridge and needs to be washed before juicing.

Juice rating: One ounce per three or four asparagus stalks.

BEETROOT

Beetroot has been cultivated since the fourth century BC and in ancient times was only used for medicinal purposes. Nowadays it is widely used as a vegetable, while it continues to have therapeutic uses. Beetroot juice is one of the most powerful cleansers and blood builders. It contains iron which builds red blood corpuscles, and although the iron content of beetroot is not particularly high, it is of a type that is easily assimilated. Because of this, beetroot juice also has a therapeutic effect on menstrual disturbances and can relieve some of the uncomfortable effects of the menopause. Beetroot juice is especially nourishing for the gall bladder, kidneys, and liver. It is high in vitamin A and so is good for both the digestive and lymphatic systems and promotes elimination of toxins. Drinking beetroot juice is also a wonderful way of adding much-needed minerals and amino acids to the diet. Since this juice is a powerful kidney and blood cleanser you may want to mix it with other juices (apple, carrot, cucumber) in case it stirs up too many toxins in one go and you could end up feeling nauseous and headachy. The dark green beet tops can be juiced as well and are packed with beta-carotene and chlorophyll.

Buying and preparing: Often beetroot is cooked before being sold, but try to buy it raw. Remove the skin before juicing.
Juice rating: Six to eight ounces per pound of beet roots or leaves.

BROCCOLI

Broccoli is a real winner when it comes to beta-carotene, which makes it a great cancer-preventing food. The American Cancer Society recommends that we eat broccoli several times a week, which it claims, 'might reduce the incidence of colon, stomach and oesophageal cancer'. Broccoli is also a rich source of vitamins C, B1 and folic acid and the minerals calcium, sulphur, iron, potassium and selenium. It has similar therapeutic properties to its relatives (cabbage, cauliflower and Brussels sprouts, etc.) and is particularly good for maintaining healthy hair, skin and eyes.
Buying and preparing: Choose bright green heads with tight tops. Yellow or brown loose heads are past their best. The stems should be firm with fresh-looking leaves; avoid woody stems. Broccoli is available throughout the year, but because it does not keep for long it should be used within one or two days. Before juicing, wash thoroughly.
Juice rating: Four to five ounces per pound of broccoli.

CABBAGE

Cabbages are thought to be the first vegetable to be cultivated and have been used for both food and medicine for thousands of years. The Greeks considered cabbages to be a wonderful tonic and rejuvenator – they even used it as a cure for baldness! Other vegetables in the cabbage (mustard) family include kale, cauliflower, Brussels sprouts and broccoli. Cabbage juice is a naturopathic favourite and often used as a cleansing tonic. It contains good amounts of vitamins A, C and E, and is rich in calcium and potassium, sulphur, phosphorus, chlorine and iodine. The combination of sulphur and chlorine has a cleansing action on the stomach and intestines. The calcium protects against osteoporosis and builds healthy bones and teeth.

Cabbage juice is an effective laxative and skin food, as well as being used for its soothing and healing effects on stomach ulcers and hiatal hernias. Dr Garnett Cheney, clinical professor at the University of California, found raw cabbage juice an effective cure for stomach ulcers. However, some people might find cabbage juice gives them wind because of its sulphur content, which reacts with the intestinal bacteria and can cause mild gas. If this happens then you can dilute the juice with water or apple or carrot juice.

Buying and preparing: Cabbages are available throughout the year and keep well in a cool place or the fridge. Look for fresh lively cabbages without damaged or wilted outside leaves. They should be washed before juicing.

Juice rating: Six ounces per pound of cabbage.

CARROT

Carrots have also been cultivated for thousands of years and will grow almost anywhere in their native Europe. They are just as happy in the sandy soil of windswept coastlines as in the relative calm of the back garden plot. British people love carrots and we eat more carrots per person than anywhere else in the world. There are over 3,000 species in the carrot (parsley) family including celery, fennel and parsnip and the herbs dill and coriander. Most of us will remember being told to eat up our carrots because they help us see in the dark, on account of their high beta-carotene content. In fact, carrots were dished up during the Second World War in aerial-training schools to improve the eyesight of the students.

It is because carrots are high in the three main antioxidant vitamins, A, C and E, that their juice often forms the basis of anti-cancer diets. According to the American cancer specialist Dr Freudenheim, 'eating a carrot a day can raise beta-carotene levels enough to give considerable protection'. Carrot juice has many other therapeutic features, including the ability to soothe and tone the intestinal walls, strengthen bones and teeth, stimulate digestion, cleanse the blood and act as a diuretic.

But perhaps its most important gift to health and beauty is in its restorative and cleansing effect on the liver. Part of the liver's job is to deal with fats and oils, and carrot juice helps to reduce fat and cholesterol levels in the blood. It also keeps our eyes bright and our skin clear. Besides containing large amounts of antioxidants, carrots also contain many of the B vitamins, calcium, iron, potassium, sodium and phosphorus.

According to Dr N W Walker, an American authority on nutrition, you can drink as many as eight pints of raw carrot juice a day. He hails it as a wonder cure for a host of illnesses because it helps normalise the entire system. It can be used to treat ulcers, intestinal and liver diseases, skin problems, sterility and cancer.

Buying and preparing: Most of the vitamins and minerals carrots contain lie just under the surface, so it is better to scrub carrots well, rather than peel them. They are available all year round and should be firm and crisp, not tired looking. If they come with their feathery tops attached, remove these quickly as they take nutrients from the roots. Carrots keep well in a cool place or in the fridge. Carrot juice gives sweetness to some of the more bitter vegetable juices and, like apple juice, makes a perfect base to almost any juice combination.

Juice rating: Six to eight ounces per pound of carrots.

CELERY

Celery has long been regarded for its healing powers and the ancient Orientals used it to cure stomach complaints and as a general tonic. The Greeks prized celery so highly, they even awarded it to their winning sportsmen.

As an all-round healthy option, celery rates highly due to its concentration of organic alkaline minerals, especially sodium.

Sodium helps to keep us young and active and our muscles limber. Natural organic sodium (not table salt which is inorganic sodium) is one of the minerals most of us lack, yet it is essential to the proper functioning of all major body systems. Organic sodium is needed by the stomach and intestines and, without sodium, good digestion is nearly impossible.

Celery juice can help to soothe digestive ailments, counteract acidosis, halt fermentation and purify the blood and lymph. One of sodium's most important jobs is to keep calcium in solution. This means that excess calcium gets eliminated from the body and is not dumped in the joints and kidneys. Celery juice helps us to make better use of our calcium and so prevents stiffness and gall- and kidney stones. It also balances the blood pH levels, preventing the build-up of acid in the joints which causes arthritis.

Celery also has important concentrations of plant hormones and essential oils which give it its distinctive smell and have the effect of regulating the brain and nervous system. The leaves can be juiced too and provide a rich source of potassium, sodium and sulphur. A combination of celery and apple juice is said to cleanse the body of excess carbon dioxide, which is good news for people living in polluted areas. As an added bonus to all celery's health-giving virtues, it is reputed to boost a flagging sex drive!

Buying and preparing: Celery stalks should be firm and crisp with fresh-looking leaves. They need to be washed before juicing and can be stored in the fridge.

Juice rating: One ounce per two or three celery stalks.

CUCUMBER

Cucumbers originally came from India where they were celebrated as a symbol of fertility. Others in the same food family include pumpkins and marrows. The old saying, 'as cool as a cucumber,' aptly describes their blood-cooling powers. On a warm day, the inside of a cucumber can be as much as twenty degrees cooler than the outside air!

They also make a wonderful digestive aid and have a cleansing effect on the bowel and skin. The high water content makes cucumber a powerful diuretic and kidney cleanser. Cucumber and carrot juice is often used for treating rheumatism as it helps to eliminate excess uric acid in the joints.

They are rich in potassium which gives elasticity to the skin cells and keeps us young looking. The high potassium content also makes them a valuable aid in controlling either high or low blood pressure. Cucumber juice is a good source of the minerals which promote healthy hair and nails – namely silicon and sulphur. Most of the vitamin A content is found in the skin of the cucumber so, as long as they are unwaxed, there is no need to peel them. If you do have to remove the skin, you can make up for the lost vitamin A by mixing in some carrot juice.

Buying and preparing: Look for unwaxed cucumbers which feel firm to touch. They need to be washed before juicing and will store well in the fridge. Cucumbers are available throughout the year.

Juice rating: Four to six ounces per pound of cucumber.

DANDELION

Most people think of dandelions as yellow-flowered weeds which clog up their lawn; however, the leaves are most nutritious and have been used for centuries as a herbal medicine. Its botanical name comes from the Greek word *taraxacum* which means 'to stir up', and French herbalists named it *dent de lion* or lion's tooth, because of its jagged leaves.

Dandelions are king of the vegetables for their vitamin A content. They are also a rich source of vitamin C, potassium, magnesium, calcium, sodium and iron. In fact they have as much iron as spinach and four times as much vitamin A as lettuce. Because of its high vitamin A content, dandelion juice is a powerful liver cleanser and helps the flow of bile. It is also thought to be an effective diuretic. A mixture of carrot and dandelion, for example, makes a perfect spring tonic and helps improve the eyesight. Magnesium is a powerful alkaliser which helps to remove acid build-up over the sedentary winter months. The magnesium content of dandelion juice also soothes and strengthens the bowel wall and the muscular and skeletal systems. The combined power of calcium and magnesium makes dandelion juice an important builder of bones and teeth. Besides this, it relieves the body of many toxic conditions that cause eczema and other skin rashes.

Buying and preparing: Dandelions are becoming more commercially available, but if you can't get them from the greengrocer, grow your own! Pick the young tender leaves which are less bitter than the mature ones. Be careful also to avoid roadside plants and any that might have been sprayed with chemicals. Dandelions taste mildest in the spring and are available until the early summer. The juice is reckoned to be one of the best spring tonics and can be sweetened with carrots and apples. Dandelion leaves will keep for a couple of days in the fridge and need to be washed before use.

Juice rating: Two ounces of juice per ten dandelion leaves.

ENDIVE (ESCAROLLE, CHICORY)

The endive is native to the East Indies. It is a curly, green, lettuce-like vegetable and is generally eaten raw in salads. It is one of the richest green vegetable sources of vitamin A, which makes it a most valuable addition to the diet, as vitamin A helps to rid the body of infections and protects against cancer.

Endive is rich in iron and potassium and makes a useful appetite stimulant because of its bitter ingredients. It is also an effective cleanser of the liver, kidneys and bladder and has been used to treat cases of hay fever and asthma and for clearing up skin problems. However, one of its main therapeutic uses is in treating eyesight defects and many people claim to have found a great improvement in their eyesight from drinking a pint or more of endive juice every day.

Endive resembles dandelion in its nutrient value and both of these are best mixed with other vegetable juices such as carrot, celery and parsley.

Buying and preparing: Buy fresh-looking green leaves. Endive needs washing before juicing. It stores well in the fridge.

Juice rating: Four to six ounces per pound of endive.

FENNEL

Fennel is an odd-looking vegetable with a distinctive and somewhat surprising aniseed flavour. It was popular in the Middle Ages, more for warding off evil spirits and witches than as a food. Nowadays, it is a well-loved salad vegetable in Italy and the French use it for treating headaches and dizziness. There are two types: garden fennel which is mainly used as a herb, and Florence fennel – a white bulb with a bright green feathery top. It's the Florence fennel that makes a lovely aromatic juice.

Since it belongs to the same family as celery, fennel shares many of the same nutrients and properties. It has an impressive content of beta-carotene, folic acid, and vitamin C and the minerals iron, calcium and magnesium. The calcium and magnesium content make fennel juice a wonderful calmer and relaxer of the nerves.

Fennel is a good blood builder and has great therapeutic effect in cases of menstrual disorders, particularly when mixed with carrot and beetroot juice.

Like celery, fennel also contains essential oils which are helpful in treating stomach upsets. A mixture of fennel and carrot juice is good for night blindness and other eye problems.

Buying and preparing: A fresh fennel bulb should be firm and white with bright green feathery leaves on top. Before juicing, discard the leaves and wash the bulb. Fennel is available throughout the year and can be stored in the fridge. It adds a pleasant flavour to other vegetable juices.

Juice rating: Six to eight ounces per pound of Florence fennel.

GINGER ROOT

Ginger root is a spice, rather than a vegetable, but merits a mention for its power to add zest and gusto to almost any juice combination.

Since ancient times ginger has been popular in the East, where it is used for both its healing properties and its pungent flavour. It is used extensively by practitioners of traditional Chinese herbal medicine and, in Japan, ginger root has been found an effective pain killer. Ginger helps to ward off colds and flu and helps to eliminate mucus from the sinuses and phlegm from the lungs. A mixture of carrot and ginger is great if you feel a cold coming on. It is also good for throat problems like laryngitis and because of its antiseptic properties ginger is especially useful in treating nausea and motion sickness. A good juice antidote for travel sickness is a combination of apple and ginger. Ginger has also been found useful in combating morning sickness.

Buying and preparing: Ginger root is a light-brown, knobbly root which should be dry and firm to touch. It is generally available throughout the year and keeps for a week or two in a cool place. You need to peel the root before juicing.

Juice rating: A piece about $1cm^3$ will add sufficient bite to most juice cocktails and gives a lovely flavour to melon and apple juice.

KALE

Kale is the oldest member of the mustard family, which includes cabbage, broccoli, cauliflower, Brussels sprouts, etc., and shares many of the same nutrients and therapeutic properties. It is particularly notable for its high calcium content and, ounce for ounce, kale juice has as much usable calcium as milk which makes it a valuable source for vegans and people with allergies to dairy products. Like others in the mustard family, kale is rich in vitamins and minerals, including sulphur which benefits the skin and hair.

Buying and preparing: Choose bright green, fresh, crisp leaves. They need to be washed before juicing. Kale is available most of the year, especially from November to May, and stores well in the fridge.

Juice rating: Six ounces of juice per pound of kale.

LETTUCE

Lettuce is one of the oldest vegetables and is thought to have originated in India or Central Asia. Both the English and Latin words for it are rooted in its milky white juice which, incidentally, contains mild sedative properties that herbalists have known about for centuries. Lettuce is both juicy and nutritious. The dark green-leaved varieties, including cos, radicchio, lamb's leaf, oakleaf and garden types, are the most nutritious. (Despite its popularity, iceberg is one of the least nutritious.)

Whatever type of lettuce you use, remember that the darker the leaves, the more nutritious it will be. The dark-leaved varieties can have up to fifty times the nutrients of the light green or white-leaved lettuces.

Lettuce is rich in calcium, magnesium, iron, potassium, silicon, vitamins A and E and chlorophyll. In particular, lettuce is a good hair and skin tonic due to its high silicon content, which adds shine and thickness to hair and a glow to the skin. Some people even claim that a glass of lettuce juice a day restores hair loss! Whether that is true or not, lettuce juice will revitalise the scalp and roots from within.

The magnesium in lettuce is exceptionally energising, particularly in the muscles, brain and nerves, and the phosphorus and sulphur content also help to calm nervous dispositions. Like most green vegetable juices, lettuce tastes better if it is mixed with other juices because it tends to be quite bitter on its own. You could mix it with carrot and spinach, for example, which will feed the nerves, hair and skin.

Buying and preparing: Lettuce should be washed well, but not left to soak as this depletes vitamins. The washing is really important. According to the US National Research Council, lettuce is one of the main sources of unwanted nitrates in our diet. To make it easier to juice leafy vegetables like lettuce, roll the leaves into balls and then push them into the juicer along with a piece of carrot or apple to help force it through.

Juice rating: Two to eight ounces per pound of lettuce. The heavier varieties make more juice than the looser-leaved types.

PARSNIP

Parsnips look a bit like pale-coloured carrots and were once the staple food of Europe's poor. They have a carbohydrate content similar to potatoes, but a nutrient value more like carrots. Parsnips are great bowel regulators and have a beneficial effect on the liver which makes them useful in detox diets. They are also mildly diuretic and anti-arthritic. Culpeper (1653) states: 'The garden parsnip nourisheth much and is good and wholesome, but a little windy. It is good for stomach and reins [kidney] and provoketh urine.'

The juice is rich in vitamin C, potassium, phosphorus, chlorine, sulphur and silicon and these latter two nutrients make it a wonderful tonic for the skin, hair and nails. It's especially good for brittle nails. Parsnip juice has also been found to be helpful to people with lung and bronchial problems; thought to be due to the combination of chlorine and phosphorus. Like carrots, parsnip juice is sweet, but it also has a distinctive nutty taste. It is a good juice for adding sweetness and flavour to bitter and less tasty vegetable juices.

Buying and preparing: Choose firm roots and store in a cool place. Parsnips need to be scrubbed before juicing.

Juice rating: Four to six ounces per pound of parsnip.

PEPPERS

Capsicum peppers belong to the *Solanaceae* family (which also includes nightshade, tobacco, potatoes, tomatoes and aubergines) and came to Europe from South and Central America. Despite coming from a potentially poisonous group of plants, peppers are a wonderfully protective food and contain many nutrients which build up resistance – notably vitamins A and C. Their rich vitamin C content compares with that found in oranges and grapefruits and helps to promote health and ward off colds.

Green peppers contain high levels of the 'beauty element' silicon which gives us healthy hair, skin, nails and teeth. It is said that fruits and vegetables with shiny skins are rich in silicon and potassium, which is certainly true in the case of peppers. This combination of nutrients not only enhances our looks but stimulates the circulation and tones and cleanses the arteries and heart.

Note: Some people are mildly affected by vegetables in the nightshade family, especially those with arthritis and joint problems who may find their condition aggravated by these foods.

Buying and preparing: The best peppers to use for juicing are the sweet or bell peppers which come in an array of bright colours – green, red, yellow, orange and black. The peppers should be smooth, firm and crisp, with a shiny skin, but if they are too shiny they have probably been waxed and these are best avoided. Peppers are available all year round. They store well in the fridge and only need a quick wash before juicing. Pepper juice is pretty strong tasting and is best diluted with other juices like tomato or carrot.

Juice rating: Four to six ounces per pound of peppers.

POTATO

Potatoes originally came from the Andean regions of tropical America – an area stretching from Chile to Mexico. They belong to the deadly nightshade family and, like their relatives, peppers and tomatoes, they were first brought to Europe after the Spanish conquest. Sir Walter Raleigh brought the first potato to England and they are now one of the world's most valuable vegetable crops. Dr Bernard Jensen, one of America's leading nutritionists says: 'I believe that if we had to confine ourselves to one food, the potato is the one on which we could live almost indefinitely.'

The humble potato is packed with minerals and vitamins, especially when eaten raw. Potato juice is a great internal cleanser and has a soothing effect on stomach ulcers and other digestive problems. It has proved successful in clearing up skin blemishes and eczema. The rich potassium content is good for the liver and kidneys, keeps the skin elastic and the muscles supple. Potassium is the body's 'healer' and is needed for rejuvenation. A combination of potato and carrot juice makes a good internal cleanser.

Potatoes are also rich in vitamin C, B vitamins, calcium, phosphorus, sulphur, chlorine and iron. In fact potatoes rank just below citrus fruits as an important source of vitamin C. Many naturopaths recommend eating some potatoes raw since many of the nutrients are lost or destroyed by cooking. Raw potatoes also contain easily digestible natural sugars, whereas cooking converts these sugars into starch.

Buying and preparing: Buy firm potatoes without any signs of damage and look for ones which have eyes, since these ones will be capable of sprouting and so will be filled with enzymes and vitality. It is important to avoid already sprouted or green potatoes because they contain a toxic substance called solanine which can cause headaches and nausea. Organic potatoes are definitely preferable because commercially grown ones tend to contain large amounts of chemical residues from pesticides, which washing cannot remove. The bulk of the nutrients lie just below the skin, therefore it is best not to peel potatoes before juicing. They need to be kept in a cool, dry, dark place.

Juice rating: Four to six ounces per pound of potatoes.

RADISH

Radishes come from the same food family as cabbages and cauliflowers and feature in ancient Egyptian records as a most popular food. There are even pictures of radishes carved on the temples at Karnak and a solid gold statue of a radish once stood in the temple at Delphi!

Radish juice is strongly diuretic and stimulates the appetite and digestion. It helps to get rid of excess mucus in the sinuses and gastrointestinal tract by its cleansing and soothing action on the mucus membranes. A mixture of radish and carrot juice is especially beneficial in this respect. Radishes are rich in vitamin C, potassium, iron and magnesium. They have a cleansing action on the kidneys, liver and gall bladder and help to break down gallstones. A juice cocktail of radish, cucumber and green pepper is especially good for cleansing these organs.

Buying and preparing: Radishes should be fresh looking, crisp and red. If they come with their green leaves attached, cut these off as soon as possible since the leaves draw the nutrients from the roots. Radishes are available throughout the year and can be stored in the fridge. The juice is very strong and is always best mixed with other juices such as carrots and cucumber.

Juice rating: Two to four ounces per pound of radishes.

SPINACH

The wonderfully rich iron content of spinach was made famous by Popeye the cartoon sailor who demonstrated Herculean feats after eating a tin of spinach. However, iron is not its only health merit; spinach is an excellent source of vitamins A, C, E, folic acid and calcium, and is about 40 percent potassium. Folic acid is especially important during pregnancy as it guards against spina bifida and anencephaly, a condition where the brain does not fully develop. Spinach revitalises the blood and is a great health restorer, and it is well known that drinking spinach juice is one of the best ways of dealing with constipation. Its potent cleansing and building properties strengthen and tone the liver, the gall bladder and the digestive, urinary and lymphatic systems.

Spinach is an extremely rich source of life-giving chlorophyll which helps to fight anaemia and fatigue.

Note: Spinach has a high oxalic acid content (especially when cooked) which combines with calcium and iron, making them difficult to absorb. For this reason many health practitioners do not rate spinach for its calcium or iron content. People with arthritis, rheumatism or gout should avoid spinach juice because its high uric acid content may aggravate their condition.

Buying and preparing: Look for crisp, fresh, bright green leaves. Spinach is widely available for about nine months of the year and can be stored for a few days in the fridge. It needs to be washed well before juicing.

Juice rating: Four to six ounces per pound of spinach.

TOMATO

Tomatoes are native to the South American Andes and were brought to Europe from Peru after the Spanish conquest. They belong to the deadly nightshade family and were initially thought to be poisonous.

Botanically, tomatoes are really fruits and have an acid content similar to oranges and grapefruits which means they have an alkalinising effect on the body. This helps to stir up toxins in the body for elimination. They are also wonderful blood and liver cleansers and form a valuable part of any detox diet. People with arthritis or gout may want to avoid tomato juice altogether or dilute it with other vegetable juices in case too many toxins are stirred up at once which will aggravate their condition. Tomatoes contain good amounts of vitamins, and are particularly high in vitamin C and beta-carotene.

Note: Tomatoes are often the cause of food intolerance and can trigger skin rashes.

Buying and preparing: Buy bright red, firm, naturally ripened tomatoes. Never use unripe, green ones as these can damage the kidneys. Organic tomatoes are definitely preferable since commercially grown ones contain high levels of pesticide residue. The US National Research Council has found that the pesticides commonly found in tomatoes have the greatest potential for causing cancer. They are available throughout the year and can be stored in the fridge.

Juice rating: Eight to ten ounces per pound of tomatoes.

TURNIP

Turnips are native to Russia, Siberia and Scandinavia. The most popular variety is the Purple-top White Globe. They are rich in beta-carotene, vitamin C, B vitamins, calcium, sulphur, iron and iodine.

The juice is especially good for any mucous or catarrhal conditions and has been successful in treating asthma and other bronchial disturbances. However, the green leaves stand out among all other vegetables for their calcium content which makes them an excellent source of this valuable mineral for young children or anyone suffering from brittle or weak bones. Ounce for ounce, turnip top juice contains more calcium than milk. For best use in the body calcium needs to have magnesium present and so it is a good idea to mix the green leaves with a magnesium vegetable like dandelion, cabbage or green peppers. For those suffering from haemorrhoids, a mixture of turnip, carrot, watercress and spinach juice is said to be a powerful cure.

Buying and preparing: Don't let the turnip tops get away because they contain 90 percent of the nutrients! The root should be firm and the leaves dark green.

Juice rating: Four to six ounces of juice per pound of turnip or per bunch of leaves.

WATERCRESS

This is another member of the mustard family (cabbage, turnips, broccoli, etc.) and thrives in watery conditions and lime soil. A native to South America, watercress has long been used in Brazil for its therapeutic effects on tuberculosis. The Romans used it as a hair tonic.

Watercress is high in the minerals and vitamins that help to ward off catarrhal conditions. It is a good blood purifier and encourages glandular secretions. It is a great health restorer and has a most beneficial effect on the digestive system, gall bladder and liver. It is a good source of the anti-cancer vitamins beta-carotene, vitamin C and vitamin E. It also provides useful amounts of folic acid, calcium, potassium, iodine and riboflavin. Watercress is a powerful cleanser and so needs to be diluted with other vegetable juices such as celery and carrot.

Apart from horseradish, watercress contains more sulphur than any other vegetable which makes it a must for healthy hair. Watercress also contains large amounts of chlorophyll which helps to oxygenate the blood and cleanse the system. It can be useful in weight-loss programmes because the juice stimulates the metabolism.

Buying and storing: Watercress leaves should be bright green and fresh looking. They need to be washed before use and can be stored in the fridge. It is available most of the year.

Juice rating: One to two ounces per bunch of watercress.

Fruit

APPLE

One of the first things we learn as children is 'A' is for apple. It is also one of the first fruits we eat. In fact, apples have been around for thousands of years and feature in many ancient legends and religious stories. Hieroglyphic writings found in the pyramids and tombs of ancient Egypt show that apples were used both as a food and as a medicine. There's an ancient Devon legend which claims that an apple rubbed on a wart will cure it! These days, there are over one thousand varieties of apple to choose from and, with summer and winter varieties, apples are available all year round. The harder, crispier ones are better for juicing. Apples are a terrific source of pectin, tannic acid and malic acid all of which remove toxins from the intestines, and regulate the bowel. The potassium and phosphorus content keeps the liver and kidneys flushed out and the skin looking good.

Apples are a good source of vitamins A and C to ward off colds and infections. They are powerful blood purifiers and benefit the blood and lymphatic systems. Apple juice is a wonderful cleanser, great for weight-reducing diets, and useful as a general tonic.

Buying and storing: Apples should be firm and crisp; avoid bruised or damaged ones. They need to be washed before juicing and should be stored in a cool, dry place. Apple juice mixes well with most other juices and can help to thin out strong-tasting juices like beetroot or thick juices like prune and strawberry.

Juice rating: Six to eight ounces per pound of apples.

APRICOT

Apricots are one of the staple foods of the remote Hunza people of the Himalayas, famed for their fitness, health and longevity. That would seem reason enough to make them a regular feature in your diet!

Apricots are the beta-carotene champions of the fruit world and therefore stand out among other fruits as cancer fighters. They help prevent cancer of the lung, oesophagus, stomach, bladder and throat, and their high vitamin C also protects against colds and flu.

Buying and preparing: Apricots have a short season and are best picked when completely ripe to ensure maximum beta-carotene content. They should be a uniform golden-orange colour and yield to slight pressure. They should be plump and juicy, not wizened, soft or mushy. Wash and stone the fruit before juicing. Apricots do not keep for long and need to be stored in a cool place.

Juice rating: Two ounces per pound of apricots.

BLACKBERRY

Blackberries are a rich source of vitamin C, with good amounts of beta-carotene, B vitamins, vitamin E, and the minerals potassium, calcium and magnesium, which makes them invaluable in cases of heart disease, cancer, high blood pressure and premenstrual tension. Blackberries also have a high iron content which makes them one of the finest blood builders. However, if you are prone to constipation you may want to mix in some prune juice to counter the possible constipating effect of the iron.

Buying and preparing: Look for plump, dark blackberries – red ones are not ripe and will not give much juice. Beware of picking roadside blackberries since fruit absorbs poisonous car exhaust fumes. Berries do not keep for long and are prone to mould so it is best to use them as soon as possible or freeze for later use. They give a wonderfully rich colour and flavour to other juices.

Juice rating: Three to four ounces per pound of blackberries.

CRANBERRY

Cranberries are native to the temperate and swampy regions of North America and Europe and like to grow on low thick vines in a bog.

Cranberry juice is commonly used for its healing properties as a natural diuretic and urinary tract cleanser. Cranberries are a rich source of vitamin C, beta-carotene, quinine, iron and potassium. The quinine helps to maintain the health of the bladder, kidneys and prostate and has been found effective in preventing prostate cancer. The high vitamin C and beta-carotene content helps to ward off cold and flu in the winter months. Cranberries have a natural antibiotic action within the body and researchers at Youngstown State University in Ohio have found that cranberry juice can prevent the rogue bacteria *Escherichia coli* from causing most urinary infections and diarrhoea. Many naturopaths use cranberry juice to treat urinary infections like cystitis and it is thought that regular drinking of cranberry juice is a good preventative measure for those prone to urinary infections. Cranberry juice tastes pretty bitter and is best sweetened with other juices such as apple or carrot.

Like citrus fruits, these berries have a heavy acid content, and so you should not drink cranberry juice too often.

Buying and preparing: Choose firm, plump berries and avoid shrivelled or damaged ones. They should be washed before juicing and can be stored in the fridge. Because cranberries are a winter fruit you can freeze them for use in the summer months.

Juice rating: Four to six ounces per pound of cranberries.

GRAPEFRUIT

Grapefruits belong to the citrus family which includes lemons, oranges, limes, tangerines, clementines and satsumas. Akin to all citrus fruits is their high vitamin C content, and grapefruits are no exception. This makes them a valuable weapon in warding off colds and infections, and helps prevent bleeding gums. Grapefruit is also a good source of beta-carotene, phosphorus, calcium and potassium. High levels of pectin, which is renowned for controlling cholesterol levels and helping with digestive problems, are found in the white pith. Bioflavonoids are found in the pith and have a protective effect on vitamin C, anti-inflammatory properties and protect the blood vessels and capillaries (see Table 1.1 for other good sources).

When using any of the citrus fruits for juicing, remember they are highly eliminative and should be used sparingly, otherwise they could stir up too many eliminations at once and leave you with skin eruptions, diarrhoea and irritated nerves! Citrus juices taken in excess can leech calcium from the bones and teeth, especially in people with lowered metabolism, such as people who are ill, the elderly and those with a sedentary lifestyle. Because they have a cleansing and nutrient value similar to oranges, grapefruits make a good alternative if oranges are causing allergic reactions.

Buying and preparing: Buy ripe, juicy grapefruits with thin skins that feel heavy for their size. The pink varieties contain up to sixteen times more beta-carotene than the more common yellow ones. They should be peeled before juicing, but be careful not to remove the nutrient-rich pith. They store well in the fridge.

Juice rating: Six to eight ounces per pound of grapefruit.

GRAPES

Grapes are one of the oldest fruits in history and are mentioned in the Bible as far back as the time of Noah. Today they are used throughout the world for their health-giving properties.

Grapes are often used in elimination and weight-loss diets because of their powerful cleansing action and their ability to stimulate the metabolism. The high magnesium content promotes good bowel movement and proper kidney function. Grape juice is also a wonderful blood and liver cleanser and eliminates unwanted uric acid from the body. Grapes are high in potassium which aids kidney function, strengthens the heart-beat and keeps the skin looking fresh and healthy.

In France, many people eat nothing but grapes during the grape season in order to cleanse the system and rebalance the body's acid/alkaline levels. In fact, studies have found a lower incidence of cancer among those who practise this annual grape diet. There are fasting clinics in Germany where grapes are frequently used as a seven-day single fruit fast with good results, especially for patients with arthritis. Dark grapes are high in iron, which makes them good blood builders.

Note: Grape juice taken on its own can be pretty sweet and so should be avoided by people with diabetes or other blood sugar disorders.

Buying and preparing: Grapes are one of the most over-sprayed crops around so it is far better to buy organic ones. Commercially grown grapes sometimes have residues of up to forty different pesticides and chemicals! Buy fresh, plump grapes for juicing and avoid overripe, shrivelled or mouldy ones that are dropping off their stems. They need to be well washed (if not organic), and can be stored in the fridge for up to a week. Don't worry about buying seedless varieties, since the seeds can go through the juicer as well. Grape juice mixes well with other juices and makes a great natural sweetener.

Juice rating: Eight ounces per pound of grapes.

KIWI

This strange-looking little fruit used to be known as a 'Chinese gooseberry', until New Zealand growers changed the name to kiwi which they thought sounded more exotic and more marketable.

In health terms, kiwis are a great source of vitamin C, containing twice as much as oranges. They are also rich in potassium which helps to reduce high blood pressure, and are good for general cleansing and warding off colds and flu. The flavour of kiwi juice has been compared to a mixture of pineapple and strawberries and it certainly helps to perk up less strong-tasting juices.

Buying and preparing: Kiwi fruit should be firm but not hard, giving to slight pressure. Imported kiwis are available all year round and can be stored for quite a while in the fridge. Peel before juicing.

Juice rating: Four to six ounces of juice per pound of kiwis.

LEMON AND LIME

Lemons and limes are probably best known for their high vitamin C content which was responsible for curing British sailors of scurvy. Long before vitamin C had been discovered, Captain Cook made sure that citrus fruits were issued to his crew – hence the nickname 'Limey' which refers to sailors who ate limes on long voyages. To bear out the wonders of citrus fruits, nearly all of Captain Cook's crews returned to shore alive in an age when just half of the crew were expected to survive a voyage.

Lemons and limes are two of the most highly alkalinising of the citrus fruits and have an exceptionally high vitamin C content. They contain up to four times the amount of citric acid as oranges or grapefruit. This high citric acid content is wonderful for getting rid of toxins; however, if the organs of elimination are not working efficiently, the process can cause uncomfortable aggravations such as constant catarrh, headaches and stiff joints.

Lemons are good for soothing sore throats and catarrhal conditions and have traditionally been used as a cure for colds and 'flu. Both fruits tend to direct eliminations through the skin, which helps heal fevers. Like grapefruit, lemons and limes are also rich in pectin and bioflavonoids.

Buying and preparing: The brighter and shinier the lemon, the more likely it is to be waxed. Try to buy unwaxed fruits with thin skins that feels heavy for their size. If not organic, lemons should be peeled before juicing, taking care to leave on the pith. They store well in the fridge.

Juice rating: Four to five ounces per pound of lemons or limes.

MANGO

Mangoes are one of the most delicious tasting fruits around and have a wonderful bright yellow juice. While we in Britain have to pay a relatively high price for them, in other regions of the world like Asia and the Caribbean they are cheap and plentiful.

Mangoes are rich in beta-carotene, vitamin C and potassium. The riper the fruit, the more beta-carotene it will contain. They are great blood cleansers and bodily disinfectants and can be effective in helping to throw off body odour.

Buying and preparing: Buy ripe mangoes which give a little when pressed, like an avocado; avoid bruised or damaged ones. Another test of freshness is their unmistakably sweet fragrance. Mangoes vary in colour from green and yellow to orange and red. Peel and remove the stone before juicing. Mangoes are tropical fruits and are best stored at room temperature.

Juice rating: Two ounces per medium-sized mango.

MELON

Melons belong to the same family as cucumbers and squash and, like cucumbers, have a cooling effect on the body. Their root systems reach deep into the soil which makes them one of the most mineral-rich fruits around.

Melons are an excellent fruit for juicing because of their high water content which makes them a first-class diuretic and wonderful kidney cleanser and skin purifier. As in many other fruits and vegetables, most of the nutrients lie in the flesh right next to the skin, so be careful not to lose this part when peeling. The juice has a light, sweet taste and mixes well with other juices. You could use it to sweeten sour juices or to dilute thick juices.

There are many varieties of melon to choose from including cantaloupe, honeydew, galia and watermelon. Cantaloupes are the most nutritious and are high in beta-carotene, vitamin C and digestive enzymes; they are highly recommended by the

American Cancer Society as a healthful agent against intestinal cancer.

Watermelons have the highest water content and are fabulous natural diuretics as well as being packed with skin-enriching minerals such as zinc and potassium.

Note: Melon ferments quickly in the stomach unless it can pass easily through the system, so melon should be eaten either alone or on an empty stomach.

Buying and preparing: Choose ripe, firm melons. As a general test, the blossom end should give slightly when ripe and they should have a pleasant aroma. Before juicing, peel the skin and remove the seeds. It is hard to tell a ripe watermelon without cutting it open, however; the flesh should be firm and juicy and with a good red colour.

Juice rating: Six to eight ounces per pound of melon.

ORANGE

Oranges are one of the oldest fruits known in history and have since become one of the most popular juices. However, all too often it is just the orange 'flavour' that is in many commercially prepared juices and little of the vitality or nutrients. Oranges are one of the richest sources of vitamin C and it is their ability to help protect against a variety of conditions from colds and flu to heart disease and strokes that gives them such a high health rating. In studies carried out by the National Cancer Institute in America, people who ate the most oranges, compared to those who ate the fewest, had the lowest incidence of developing cancer. As an antioxidant, vitamin C helps to mop up damaging free radicals which age the skin and cause premature wrinkles and sagging. You need to peel the fruit before juicing, being careful to leave on the pith, since this is where most of the nutrients are, including vitamins C and A and the B-complex vitamins, bioflavonoids, pectin, amino acids, potassium, zinc and phosphorus.

Vitamin C helps iron to be better absorbed in the body, so a glass of orange juice a day can actually double the amount of iron available for use in the body. The high citric acid content in oranges is most effective in cleansing the gastrointestinal tract and eliminating toxins and acid wastes in the cells. For this reason, orange juice is often included in eliminative diets.

Vitamin C and bioflavonoids act as anticoagulants, strengthen the blood vessels and capillaries and ward off colds and flu. Both the heart and lungs benefit from regular drinking of orange juice. It's always a good idea to increase your supply of vitamin C in the winter months, and what better way than by drinking a glass of fresh juice.

Buying and preparing: Look for firm, heavy oranges with bright, fresh looking skin. Avoid ones with damaged or wrinkled dry skin. Oranges are available throughout the year and keep well in a cool place.

Juice rating: Six to eight ounces per pound of oranges.

PAPAYA

The one thing that distinguishes papaya from other fruit is its incredible digestive properties. Papayas are rich in papain, a protein-digesting enzyme, which is so effective that it is used in meat tenderisers and digestants. The juice has a marvellous effect on stomach ulcers and fevers and many people have hailed papayas as the great rejuvenator, combating premature ageing. This may be due to the fact that poor digestion leads to malnourished cells, while efficient digestion ensures that the cells are properly fed.

Papaya juice makes a valuable digestive aid and has been known to correct stomach upsets extremely quickly. As early as the 1930s doctors were using papain to treat allergies. Because it improves the body's ability to digest food properly, papain increases allergic tolerance. Papaya mixes well with pineapple, which also contains digestive enzymes. If you are using papaya primarily for its digestive properties, buy it when it is still green and unripe as unripe papayas have much more active papain than ripe ones.

Another plus point for papayas is their ability to restore a healthy balance of intestinal bacteria after the use of antibiotics. Papaya juice also strengthens the body's coagulating ability. It makes an effective laxative and cleanser of the liver, kidneys and intestines and has the ability to dissolve excess mucus in the body.

Papayas are especially rich in beta-carotene, vitamins C and E, and the minerals calcium, phosphorus and iron.

Buying and preparing: Papayas are sometimes called pawpaws. Ripe papayas are an orange/yellow colour and give a little when squeezed. Before juicing, cut them in half and scoop out the flesh. **Juice rating:** One to three ounces per pound of papaya.

PEACH

Peaches have been cultivated for over four thousand years and are thought to have originally come from China. If conditions are right, a peach tree can live for hundreds of years. Peaches, like other yellow-coloured fruits, are an excellent source of beta-carotene. They also contain vitamin C, some of the B vitamins, and minerals such as calcium, iron, phosphorus, potassium and sodium.

Peach juice is wonderfully alkalinising and cleanses the intestinal tract and encourages good bowel movement. Drinking peach juice will improve your skin and eyesight and help prevent against cancer and heart disease. It has often been used by pregnant women to prevent morning sickness.

Buying and preparing: Choose ripe, unbruised peaches and avoid overripe, green or damaged ones. To prepare – wash well, cut in half and remove the stone. Peach juice is fairly thick and can be thinned out with other juices like apple and orange. **Juice rating:** One to three ounces per pound of peaches. The riper the peach, the more juice it will yield.

PEAR

Pears are native to Europe and are available all year round in one variety or another. Common to all pears is their sweetness and this makes them ideal for mixing with the more bitter juices.

They have a high content of vitamin C and B vitamins and the minerals potassium, phosphorus and iron. Pear juice is a wonderful digestive aid and helps to normalise the bowel. It is a valuable addition to elimination diets because of its mild diuretic and laxative effect. In fact, pear juice is one of the best urinary and gastrointestinal cleansers because of its high level of pectin.

Buying and preparing: Buy pears which are still firm to the touch and avoid overripe or bruised ones. Overripe pears may clog up your juicer and do not provide as much juice. Pears can be kept in the fridge for up to a week. Before juicing, wash the outside well and split into quarters.

Juice rating: Four to six ounces per pound of pears.

PINEAPPLE

Pineapples are native to tropical America and were highly rated among the discoveries of Columbus. Nowadays, they are grown all over the world and can be bought throughout the year.

Because of their high vitamin C content pineapples are considered to be a protective fruit. The juice is wonderful for relieving constipation and poor digestion and the combination of vitamin C, fruit acids and enzymes makes pineapples highly eliminative and a great boost for detox diets.

Pineapples contain the digestive enzyme bromelin which, like the enzymes in papaya, breaks down protein and dissolves excess mucus. In fact, bromelin can digest one thousand times its weight of protein. It is so strong that workers in canning factories have to wear protective gloves to stop their skin from being eaten away by the juice. Bromelin also balances the body's acid/alkaline levels, soothes sore throats and has been found to cure laryngitis.

Other nutrients found in pineapples include beta-carotene, folic acid, potassium, iodine, calcium and magnesium.

Buying and preparing: Pineapples should have a golden-coloured skin and smell strong and sweet. Supposedly, the ultimate test of ripeness is whether you can pull a leaf off the stem easily – if not, then it is not ripe. Before juicing, remove the spiny top and, unless organic, pineapples should also be peeled. All the flesh and the core can be juiced. They should be stored at room temperature when whole and in the fridge if cut into pieces.

Juice rating: Four to six ounces per pound of pineapple.

PRUNES

Prunes are a variety of dried plums and are widely used as a natural laxative. Prune juice is just as potent as the whole fruit and is a much healthier way to treat constipation than using synthetic laxatives.

Buying and preparing: It is best to buy prunes which are not oiled or preserved with sulphur dioxide and which are already pitted. To get the most out of prunes, soak them overnight in warm water and juice them the following day. The juice is quite thick but can be diluted with apple, for example, to make a potent laxative.

Juice rating: Varies depending how much water is used for soaking.

RASPBERRY

Raspberries are good cleansers – especially of mucous and catarrhal conditions. They are natural astringents and can help sort out upset stomachs, bowel problems and gum disease. Raspberries are high in vitamins A and C and provide useful amounts of potassium, calcium and magnesium which makes them invaluable in cases of heart problems, fatigue or depression. The juice has a wonderful flavour and gives a rich colour to other juice combinations. A raspberry-juice cocktail before meals stimulates the appetite and aids digestion.

Buying and preparing: Choose fresh, plump berries that are not damaged or mushy. Raspberries are a summer fruit and do not keep for long, although they can be frozen and used during the winter months.

Juice rating: Four ounces per pound of raspberries.

STRAWBERRY

Strawberries are native to the Americas and are a wonderful source of vitamin C, beta-carotene, potassium, calcium and iron.

They are cleansing and eliminative which makes them a great spring cleaner. They have also been found to relieve arthritis, and the renowned Swedish botanist Linnaeus cured his own arthritis by fasting on strawberries. Because of their high sodium content they can also be considered a 'youthful' food and their high potassium content is good for the skin. The high levels of beta-carotene and vitamin C help to fight off colds and infections, and to prevent cancer and heart disease. Potassium and iron help to strengthen the blood. Strawberry is also one of the few fruit juices that contain natural pain killers, some of which form the basis of synthetic drugs like aspirin.

Strawberry juice is fairly thick and sweet and is best diluted with other juices or used to flavour less strong-tasting juices.

Buying and preparing: Locally grown strawberries are widely available in the summer months and are preferable to imported fruits which may contain high amounts of chemical residue or which may have been irradiated. They should be plump, firm and bright red with the green top still on. They need to be washed before juicing and can be stored for a few days in the fridge; however, it is worth noting that the vitamin C content diminishes the longer they are stored.

Juice rating: Four to five ounces per pound of strawberries.

WATERMELON – *SEE MELON*

Sprouted Seeds and Beans, Herbs and Wheatgrass

Although sprouted seeds and beans, wheatgrass and herbs are not covered in detail in this book, do experiment with them since they are a terrific source of nutrients.

Sprouted seeds and beans are easy to grow, and guaranteed organic if you do it yourself! It's also fun watching the little seeds or beans burst into life in a matter of days. There is a variety of seeds or beans you could try, like alfalfa, adzuki, sesame, mung and chickpea.

Herbs are also a most valuable addition to juicing. Parsley, for example, is a rich source of vitamin C and iron, and nettles and dandelions are wonderful cleansers and diuretics.

Growing your own wheatgrass is a bit more of an undertaking than herbs and sprouted seeds and beans but nevertheless is worth every effort. Wheatgrass is a wonderful source of life-giving enzymes, chlorophyll and other essential nutrients, and many naturopaths advocate it in cancer treatment.

If you do wish to branch out beyond fruit and vegetable juices there are plenty of good books on sprouted seeds and beans, herbs and wheatgrass to help you along. You may also want to get one of the juicers more suited to extracting juice from tough fibrous material, such as the Health Fountain Juicer (see page 23).

Unjuiceables

Some fruit and vegetables fall into the unjuiceable category mainly because it is hard to extract the juice from the pulp, like avocados and bananas. Rhubarb is best left alone because it contains a high amount of oxalic acid.

5

Juice Cures

The focus of health care has changed rapidly over the past ten to fifteen years as more and more people are beginning to understand that symptoms of disease are outward signs of a *general* lack of harmony and balance in their lives.

Practitioners of natural medicine prescribe health-building lifestyles, rather than drugs, which help to cleanse and strengthen the body from within, so that it can self-heal and protect itself against potentially damaging diseases such as heart disease and cancer. In her book *A Time to Heal*, Beata Bishop describes her fight against cancer and her eventual recovery after following the Gerson Therapy diet and re-evaluating her entire lifestyle and outlook. American 'Juiceman' Jay Korvich has a favourite juice which is simply a mixture of apple and carrot, which he believes saved his life. You too can reap the benefits of nature's treasury by incorporating fresh fruit and vegetable juices into your daily diet.

This chapter lists in alphabetical order some of the most common complaints and their recommended juice recipes. It is generally agreed that you need to drink at least one pint per day of your chosen juice for a number of weeks to effect a change. (The following list of ailments and juice recommendations is only a *guide* and shouldn't be regarded as a cure-all. Anyone with a serious disease should always consult a doctor or an experienced healthcare practitioner.)

There are several fruit and vegetable juices listed for each ailment, but this is just a guide – the rest is up to you! However, carrot juice has been shown to have the most wide-ranging effects on health and makes a great base for almost any other vegetable or fruit combination.

AILMENT	RECOMMENDED JUICES
Anaemia	Apple, asparagus, beetroot, blackberry, carrot, celery, dandelion, fennel, black grape, lettuce, parsley, prune, spinach, strawberry, turnip, watercress.
Antibiotics	(ie after treatment with) Apple, cranberry, cucumber, garlic, onion, papaya.
Arthritis	Apple, carrot, celery, cucumber, fennel, grape, grapefruit, parsnip, potato, spinach, strawberry, turnip.
Asthma	Carrot, endive, parsnip, radish, spinach,turnip.
Bad breath	Apple, carrot, cucumber, lemon, spinach.
Bladder disorders	Beetroot, cabbage, carrot, cucumber, dandelion, endive, parsnip, spinach, watercress.
Blood pressure (high)	Beetroot, cabbage, carrot, cucumber, kiwi, orange, papaya, parsley, pineapple, spinach.
Blood pressure (low)	Beetroot, carrot, celery, cucumber, spinach, watercress.
Bones and teeth	Broccoli, cabbage, carrot, dandelion, kale, parsnip, tomato, turnip, turnip top.
Cancer	Apricot, asparagus, beetroot, blackberry, blackcurrant, broccoli, carrot, celery, endive, grape, kiwi, mango, melon, orange, peach, potato, radish, spinach, strawberry, turnip, watercress.

Catarrh	Beetroot, carrot, celery, cucumber, ginger, radish, raspberry, spinach, turnip, watercress.
Colds	Apricot, carrot, ginger, grapefruit, kiwi, lemon, lime, orange, pepper, pineapple, potato, strawberry, tomato.
Colitis	Apple, beetroot, cabbage, carrot, cucumber, papaya, spinach.
Constipation	Apple, cabbage, carrot, lettuce, papaya, peach, pear, pineapple, prune, spinach.
Cystitis	Cranberry, pear.
Diabetes	Asparagus, Brussels sprout, carrot, celery, endive, lettuce, parsley, spinach.
Digestive system	Beetroot, carrot, celery, cucumber, endive, grapefruit, lemon, papaya, pear, pineapple, radish, raspberry, watercress.
Eye trouble	Asparagus, beetroot, broccoli, carrot, celery, cucumber, dandelion, endive, fennel, parsley, peach, spinach, turnip.
Fatigue	Beetroot, carrot, lemon, lettuce, orange, raspberry, spinach, watercress.
Fatty degeneration	Beetroot, carrot, cucumber, spinach.
Fever	Celery, cucumber, grape, grapefruit, lemon, lime, orange.
Fluid retention	Asparagus, carrot, cranberry, cucumber, dandelion, melon, parsnip, pear, radish, watermelon.
Gall bladder and gallstones	Apple, beetroot, carrot, celery, cucumber, dandelion, radish, spinach, watercress.

Gout	Apple, beetroot, carrot, celery, fennel, lemon, lime, orange, parsley, pineapple, spinach.
Haemorrhoids (piles)	Apple, carrot, grape, pear, potato, spinach, turnip, watercress.
Hair	Asparagus, broccoli, cabbage, carrot, cucumber, kale, lettuce, parsnip, pepper, watercress.
Hay fever	Beetroot, carrot, celery, endive, kale, parsnip, spinach.
Headaches	Apple, beetroot, cabbage, carrot, celery, fennel, spinach.
Heart disease	Beetroot, blackberry, carrot, dandelion, endive, papaya, pepper, pineapple, raspberry, spinach, strawberry.
Hernia	Cabbage, carrot, celery, cucumber, parsley, spinach.
Indigestion	Beetroot, cabbage, carrot, cucumber, lettuce, papaya, peach, pineapple, spinach, tomato.
Insomnia	Carrot, celery, lettuce.
Kidney disorders	Apple, asparagus, beetroot, broccoli, cabbage, carrot, celery, cranberry, cucumber, endive, grape, melon, potato, watermelon.
Liver disorders	Apple, asparagus, beetroot, carrot, celery, dandelion, endive, grape, grapefruit, kale, lemon, lime, papaya, parsnip, pear, potato, spinach, watercress.
Lymph circulation	Apple, beetroot, celery.

Menstrual problems	Beetroot, fennel, watercress.
Morning sickness	Ginger, peach.
Nails	Cucumber, parsnip, pepper.
Nervous system	Asparagus, carrot, celery, fennel, lettuce, spinach.
Pregnancy	Beetroot, carrot, cucumber, dandelion, grapefruit, kale, lettuce, parsley, parsnip, peach, spinach, turnip, watermelon.
Premenstrual tension	Blackberry.
Prostate trouble	Asparagus, beetroot, carrot, cranberry, lemon, lettuce, pear, spinach.
Rheumatism	Apple, asparagus, beetroot, carrot, celery, cucumber, grape, lemon, orange, strawberry.
Sexual drive	Asparagus, beetroot, carrot, celery, cucumber, watercress.
Skin disorders	Apple, asparagus, beetroot, broccoli, cabbage, carrot, dandelion, endive, grape, grapefruit, kale, lettuce, lime, melon, orange, parsnip, pepper, potato, radish, spinach, strawberry, tomato, turnip, watercress, watermelon.
Throat problems	Carrot, ginger, lemon, lime, pineapple.
Travel sickness	Apple, ginger.
Ulcers	Beetroot, cabbage, carrot, papaya, potato, spinach.

Viral infections	Carrot, celery, citrus fruits, garlic, parsley, pineapple.
Varicose veins	Asparagus, beetroot, carrot, celery, grapefruit, parsley, potato, spinach.
Weight loss	Apple, beetroot, carrot, celery, cucumber, dandelion, endive, fennel, grape, grapefruit, lemon, lettuce, lime, orange, papaya, parsnip, pineapple, radish, spinach, tomato, watercress, watermelon.

——6——

Inner Cleansing
Juice Diet

The only way to inner cleanse is by removing toxins from the body. And the best way to cleanse is by fasting, either on water alone or on juices. Juices are nature's cleansers and whether drunk alone or combined with solid food they make a huge difference to the way we look and feel. This chapter provides recipe ideas for juice fasting and a healthy eating plan for an all-round cleansing diet.

Inner cleansing through detoxification has been going on for thousands of years and anything that has been going on for that long must have something going for it! A period of detoxification lets the body cleanse and renew and most people feel great after even a short detox. Toxins are nothing new – they have been around for as long as fasting and are formed as natural byproducts of the digestive processes, such as uric acid, lactic acid and adrenalin. However, if the body gets overburdened with waste products, it cannot efficiently eliminate these natural toxins, let alone deal with the unnatural toxins we take in from chemicals and other environmental pollutants. In today's world excess wastes and impurities build up in the body, which leads to slow metabolism, sluggishness, fatigue, skin blemishes, dull hair and eyes and general malaise. All these things are telling us that we need to inner cleanse. A healthy system can cope with a certain amount of toxins, but when we bombard it with too much salt, alcohol, cigarette smoke, stress, worry, food allergies, frustration, anger, chemicals, lack of exercise and bad diet then we can't cope and our body begins to complain.

A JUICE DETOX PLAN HELPS TO:

* rid the body of accumulated wastes by releasing them from the cells and tissues
* flush waste products out through the kidneys, liver, lungs, skin and colon
* restore the right pH balance
* strengthen the blood and immune systems
* give the body a rest.

The outward signs of an inner cleanse are glowing skin, shiny hair, sparkling eyes, vitality, zest and much more!

How Often Should You Detox?

It really depends on what you can manage individually and what commitments and lifestyle you have. At the very least though, most healthy people can manage a one-day juice fast and the American 'Juiceman' Jay Korvich recommends juice fasting one day every week. Longer fasts of three days can be done monthly or so. We all need regular cleansing. Common ailments like allergies, mood swings, headaches, depression and skin problems occur when the body is clogged up and under strain. The idea behind any inner cleansing diet is also educational. Eventually your body will be re-educated into new and healthier ways of eating and a healthier lifestyle.

Weight Loss

Fresh juices are great for any weight-loss programme since they are virtually fat free, low in calories and high in nutrients. For example an 8oz glass of fruit juice contains about 100 calories, and the same amount of vegetable juice contains even less than that. Juices also help to curb the appetite and speed up the metabolism. Any plan of healthy eating will tend to 'normalise' the whole system and bring you to your personal optimum weight. A short juice fast can be a step in the right direction, but any permanent weight loss requires permanent changes in the way you eat and live.

Cellulite

Cellulite is really a build-up of toxins in the fat cells. Nature is wise and puts toxins in the least harmful areas, away from vital organs and tissues like the heart and brain. Fat cells are a relatively safe place to dump toxins, but cellulite is still a sign that the body could do with a detox. Banishing cellulite is an ongoing campaign in which juice fasts play a valuable role. Any health gains take time and effort and a willingness to change. If you think about it, we are today what we ate yesterday, and only you can change that.

One-Day Juice Fast

GETTING READY

* It is important to get ready *mentally* which means getting into a positive frame of mind so that you can complete the fast.
* Set aside a day when you can relax and rest as much as possible as this will benefit your whole system. You may want to book a massage appointment or a sauna on that day to assist with the cleansing process.
* Make sure you have all the ingredients you will need for the fast day – including fruit and vegetables, herb teas, etc. and optional extras such as dry skin brush, Epsom salts or enema kit (see page 76).

* It is also a good idea to keep as quiet and peaceful as possible, avoiding television and busy places. Cleansing is a time to look inward and peace and quiet will help tremendously.

* Prepare your digestive system the day before the fast. This can be a mono-fruit day or just eating lightly, avoiding meat, fish, eggs, dairy produce and wheat. The most powerful juice fast is a fruit juice fast, since juices are stronger cleansers than vegetables, especially citrus fruit. However, a pure fruit juice fast could stir up too many toxins at once and leave you feeling a bit rough. Ideally, try to drink a mix of fruit and vegetable juices throughout the day plus plenty of filtered or bottled water and herb teas if desired.

SHOPPING LIST:

4 apples
8 carrots
1/4 cucumber
1 celery stick
2 oranges
1 lemon
Some fresh root ginger
Bottled or filtered water
Selection of herb teas
Optional:
Vegetable bristle body brush
Enema kit and freshly ground organic coffee
1–2lbs Epsom salts
Psyllium husks

THE TIMETABLE

On rising	A glass of warm water with a squeeze of lemon juice and/or ginger. This helps cleanse the intestines and restore the pH balance. Body brush, shower, do some light exercise like yoga or breathing exercises.
Breakfast	8–10oz glass of apple, orange and ginger juice (see page 78).
Mid-morning	8–10oz glass water or a herb tea.
Lunch	8–10oz glass of carrot and apple juice (see page 80).
Afternoon	8–10oz glass of water or a herb tea.
Supper	8–10oz glass of carrot, celery and cucumber juice (see page 80).
Evening	8–10oz glass of water or a herb tea.
Before bed	8–10oz glass of warm water with a squeeze of lemon juice and/or ginger

Try to drink about 1–2 litres of filtered or bottled water as well as the juices to help flush toxins out of the system.

Three juices per day will probably be enough to start with since they are powerful cleansers and can stir up toxins faster than you can comfortably eliminate. You can also dilute juices with water if you feel they may be too strong. If you want to have more than three juices a day then using enemas, psyllium husks or Epsom salt baths will really help with elimination (see page 76 for details).

Any detox programme is greatly enhanced if you also take some light exercise such as yoga, walking or breathing exercises, but remember not to overdo it, since the body needs all its energy for cleansing and you could feel slightly weak or faint if you don't take it easy. Relaxation is an important part of detox diets. This is also a perfect time to pamper yourself – have a massage, a sauna or a facial, for example. You could use the time to read, write letters, sew, meditate or listen to music.

Three-Day Fast

Follow the guidelines for the one-day fast for three consecutive days. You can choose different juices for each 'meal' from the Recipes chapter, or make up your own. The longer you fast, the greater the depth of cleansing. The body has more time in which to surrender its toxins for clearing and for rebuilding worn and damaged tissues.

The first day is always the hardest because the body needs time to adapt to going without food and you may feel a little hungry. But the rewards are great and you will have much more energy and clarity of mind after fasting. Because more toxins will be dug out of the cells on a longer fast you may feel slightly unwell as the toxins are released into the system for clearing. Naturopaths may recommend including enemas, Epsom salt baths, or psyllium husks during the three fast days to help with elimination (see pages 75–6). Caffeine enemas are reputed to be especially good at stimulating the liver and helping it to detoxify through the bowel.

DAILY ELEMENTS OF A FAST:
* *Diet* – Fresh juices, bottled or filtered water, herb teas.
* *Internal cleansing* – enemas, psyllium husks.
* *External cleansing* – Epsom salts, sauna, steam bath, skin brushing, shower.
* *Exercise* – walking, swimming, cycling, yoga, breathing, t'ai chi, stretch, rebounding.
* *Rest.*
* *Peace.*

Optional Extras

These are by no means essential to cleansing and detoxification but they can help to eliminate toxins from the body. Years of bad eating habits and sluggish organs of elimination can lead to a build-up of toxins which is particularly hard to shift through juicing alone. These optional extras are designed to thoroughly cleanse and stimulate our organs of detoxification such as the skin and the bowel. However, it is always better to consult your doctor or health care practitioner first if you are at all unsure about any of the following aids to elimination.

PSYLLIUM HUSKS

Psyllium husks, the seeds of the plaintain, are a form of natural fibre and are unsurpassed in their ability to remove sticky mucus and toxins from the bowel. They can be taken as capsules or stirred loose into water. The important thing is to ensure that you drink at least one glass of water per three or four capsules or teaspoon of husks. This is because they swell up with water to form a bulky jelly-like mass which absorbs toxins and carries them out of the body. Psyllium husks are a well-known remedy for ulcers and constipation, they reduce acidity and increase urine flow. A similar effect can also be achieved with linseeds. The husks are available in most health-food stores and make a great addition to any detox or cleansing diet.

LINSEEDS

Linseeds are rich in fibre and essential fatty acids and can be used instead of psyllium husks. Take one desertspoon of linseeds two or three times daily with one of your juices or some live yoghurt, or sprinkle them on soups and salads. For the seeds to work effectively, it is important that you drink at least 1/4 pint (150ml) per desertspoon of seeds.

DRY SKIN BRUSHING

Brushing your skin all over with a dry brush may sound a little odd, but it is a great way to stimulate the lymphatic system and it clears and revitalises the skin. Use a vegetable bristle brush on dry skin, brush the body in brisk sweeps towards the lower abdomen. You always begin at the feet and move upwards until you reach the abdomen, then begin to brush down from the neck and shoulders. Body brushes are fairly easy to get hold of from chemists and health-food stores.

EPSOM SALT BATHS

Epsom salts are made from magnesium sulphate and they draw impurities from the skin. Add about 1–2lbs of salts to a hot bath and soak for fifteen to twenty minutes. When you get out, wrap yourself up in warm clothes, get into bed and sweat, sweat, sweat! As you perspire toxins will be eliminated through the skin. Epsom salts are available from chemists and some health-food stores.

ENEMAS

Coffee enemas help to stimulate the liver and encourage detoxification through the bowel. (Drinking coffee doesn't have this same beneficial effect!) To prepare a coffee enema, put three tablespoons of real ground, organic coffee into a pint of water and let it boil for three minutes and then simmer for a further fifteen minutes. Strain and use at body temperature. Make the liquid up to about two pints before use. Always lie on your right side with your knees up to your chest when doing an enema and try to keep the liquid in for fifteen to twenty minutes. If you find you can only manage to keep it in a short while, then use less liquid and halve the strength. You can buy enemas kits from chemists and suppliers of health products.

—7—

Recipes

The Juices

There are hundreds of juice combinations that can be made – all it takes is a little imagination! The following recipes are a guide to start you off. They are split into three groups – fruit juices, vegetable juices and green juices. The main thing to remember is that, with the exception of carrot and apple juice, vegetable juices and fruit juices shouldn't be mixed or you may experience flatulence and bloating. Fruit juices are best taken in the earlier part of the day since they are basically cleansing foods, highly eliminative and good energisers. Their high water content flushes toxins from the digestive tract, kidneys and bloodstream. Citrus fruits are strong solvents and shouldn't be taken in large quantities by people with lowered or impaired digestion. The green vegetable juices are more calming and give long-term energy which makes them a great evening drink. Whatever your preference, do try to get a varied mix of fruit and vegetable juices in the course of the day so that you can reap the maximum benefits of nature's garden and the full range of nutrients.

The following recipes will each make approximately 8–10oz of fresh juice. Unless you are using organic fruit and vegetables, all produce should be peeled before juicing.

FRESH FRUIT JUICES
Apple and orange
2 apples
2 oranges
Wash and slice the apples, peel the oranges, leaving the pith. Juice.

Apple, orange and ginger
2 apples
2 oranges
2cm cube of fresh ginger
Wash and slice the apples, peel the ginger, peel the oranges, leaving the pith. Juice.

Apple, pineapple and pear
1 medium apple
1/3 pineapple
2 pears
Wash and slice the apple and pears, peel the pineapple. Juice.

Apple, orange and strawberry
2 apples
1 orange
1/2lb strawberries
Wash and slice the apples, peel the orange and wash and hull the strawberries. Juice.

Apple and grape
2 apples
1/2lb grapes
Wash the fruit, remove the grapes from the stem, slice the apple. Juice.

Apple, pear (and cranberry)
2 medium apples
1 pear
1/2lb cranberries – if you can't get hold of cranberries you can make up the quantity by using another pear.
Wash the fruit, slice the apples and pear. Juice.

Apple, orange and apricot
2 apples
1 orange
6 apricots
Wash and slice the apples and apricots, peel the orange. Juice.

Kiwi, apple and green grape
2 kiwi fruits
1 apple
1/2lb green grapes
Wash the fruit, peel the kiwis, slice the apple. Juice.

Orange, grapefruit and lemon (or lime)

2 oranges
1 grapefruit
1 lemon/lime
Peel all fruit. Juice.

Apple, raspberry (and mango)

2 apples
1/2lb raspberries
1 mango – if mangoes are not in season use another apple instead.
Wash the raspberries, wash and slice the apples, peel and stone the mango. Juice.

Orange, peach (and mango)

2 oranges
2 peaches
1 mango – if mangoes are not in season use another peach instead.
Wash and stone the peaches, peel and stone the mango, peel the oranges. Juice.

Apple, pineapple (and papaya)

1 apple
1/2 pineapple
1 papaya – if you can't get hold of a papaya, use another apple instead.
Wash and slice the apple, halve the papaya and scoop out the flesh, peel the half pineapple. Juice.

Melon mix

1/4 honeydew melon
1 slice of watermelon
1/2 galia melon
Peel the melons, remove the seeds. Juice.

Apple, carrot, melon and ginger

1 apple
2 carrots
1/2 galia melon
1cm cube of fresh ginger
Peel the melon and scoop out the seeds, wash the other ingredients, trim the carrots, peel the ginger. Juice.

Apple, grapefruit and pineapple
1 apple
1 grapefruit
1/2 pineapple

Wash and slice the apple, peel the grapefruit, leaving the pith, cut the rind off the pineapple. Juice.

Apple and prune
2 apples
6 prunes (soaked overnight in 6oz water)

Wash and peel the apples, pit the prunes. Juice using the prune water as well.

Apple and black grape or blackberry
2 apples
1/2lb black grapes or 1/2lb blackberries

Wash the fruit, slice the apples. Juice.

FRESH VEGETABLE JUICES

Here are a few vegetable juice ideas to get you going. You may want to begin with your favourite ones first before branching out into new and unusual flavours.

Carrot and apple
4 medium carrots
2 medium apples

Wash and slice the apples, wash and trim the carrots. Juice. Carrot and apple gives a perfect base to almost any fresh juice combination.

Carrot, apple and ginger
4 carrots
2 apples
1cm cube of fresh ginger

Wash and slice the apples, wash and trim the carrots, peel the ginger. Juice.

Carrot, celery and cucumber
  4 carrots
  1/3 cucumber
  1 celery stick
Wash and trim the vegetables.
Juice.

Carrot, cucumber and beetroot
  4 carrots
  1/4 cucumber
  1/2 beetroot
Wash and trim all the
vegetables. Juice.

Carrot, apple and watercress
  4 carrots
  2 apples
  Few sprigs of watercress
Wash all the ingredients, trim
the carrots, slice the apples.
Juice. (Use the carrots to push
the watercress through the
juicer.)

Carrot, apple and red cabbage
  4 carrots
  1 apple
  1/4lb red cabbage
Wash the ingredients, trim the
carrots, slice the apple. Juice.

Carrot, fennel and cucumber
  3 carrots
  1/2 fennel bulb
  1/4 cucumber
Wash and trim the vegetables,
slice the cucumber and fennel.
Juice.

Carrot, apple, green pepper and celery
  3 carrots
  1 apple
  1/2 green pepper
  1 celery stick
Wash all the ingredients, trim
the carrots and celery, slice the
apples, de-seed the pepper.
Juice.

Tomato, red pepper and cucumber
  1/2lb tomatoes
  1/2 red pepper
  1/4 cucumber
Wash the ingredients, slice the
tomatoes, and cucumber,
de-seed the red pepper. Juice.

Carrot, tomato and beetroot
  2 carrots
  5 tomatoes
  1/2 beetroot
Wash the ingredients, trim the
carrots, peel the beetroot. Juice.

Carrot, celery and parsnip

4 carrots
1 celery stick
1 medium parsnip

Wash and trim the parsnip, carrots and celery. Juice.

Apple, carrot, celery and lettuce

2 apples
2 carrots
6 lettuce leaves
1 celery stick

Wash the ingredients, trim the celery, slice the apples. Juice. (It is easier to juice leafy vegetables if you roll the leaves into tight balls and then push them through the juicer with a piece of hard vegetable.)

Carrot, radish and spinach

4 carrots
6 radishes
Handful of spinach

Wash the ingredients, trim the carrots and radishes. Juice.

Carrot, cabbage, celery and fennel

2 carrots
1/4 head of cabbage
1 celery stick
1/2 fennel bulb

Wash ingredients, trim the fennel and carrots. Juice.

Fennel and apple

1/2 fennel bulb
3 apples

Wash and slice the ingredients. Juice.

Carrot, tomato (and dandelion or parsley)

4 tomatoes
4 carrots
6 dandelion leaves or small bunch of parsley

Wash the ingredients, trim the carrots. Juice.

Carrot, beetroot and parsley

5 carrots
1/2 beetroot
Few sprigs of parsley

Wash and trim the carrots, peel the beetroot. Juice.

Carrot and spinach

6 carrots
Handful of spinach

Wash the ingredients well, trim the carrots. Juice.

Fresh Green Juices

Apple, green pepper and lettuce

3 apples
1/2 green pepper
6 lettuce leaves

Wash the ingredients, slice apples, core and de-seed pepper. Juice.

Apple, cucumber and spinach

3 apples
1/4 cucumber
6 spinach leaves

Wash the vegetables, trim the cucumber, slice the apple. Juice.

Apple, broccoli and lettuce

2 apples
1/2lb broccoli
6–8 lettuce leaves

Wash all the ingredients, slice the apples, trim the broccoli. Juice.

Apple, kale, parsley and cucumber

2 apples
4oz kale
Few sprigs of parsley
1/4 cucumber

Wash the ingredients, slice the apple. Juice.

Apple, asparagus and watercress

2 apples
4 asparagus stalks
Handful of watercress

Wash the ingredients, trim the asparagus, slice the apples. Juice.

Cabbage, apple and celery

1/4 head of green cabbage
2 apples
1 celery stick

Wash the ingredients, slice the apples, trim the celery. Juice.

Juicing is fun! and with a little imagination you can make up hundreds of different recipes. The thing to remember is that both carrot and apple juice make wonderful foundations for almost any other juice combination and you can almost go on for ever building new juices from this foundations. Variety is the key to health and this goes for juices too. In fact, variety itself may be the best protection against nutritional deficiencies because different vegetables and fruits contain different ratios of key nutrients. Start by making your favourite flavours and build up to more adventurous tastes. For example ...

Carrot
Apple
Carrot + apple
Carrot + orange
Carrot + lettuce
Carrot + cucumber
Carrot + apple + pear
Carrot + apple + celery
Carrot + apple + pineapple
Carrot + apple + lettuce + pepper
Carrot + apple + raspberry + orange
Carrot + apple + raspberry + strawberry ...

Soups

Fresh juices can also be incorporated into tasty recipes to boost the flavour and nutritional value of food. Try these delicious soup recipes before experimenting with your own ideas.

Carrot and cashew soup

225g (1/2lb) onions
2 cloves garlic
450g (1lb) carrots
Juice of 1/2 lemon
100g (4oz) cashew nuts
30ml (2tbsp) olive oil
5ml (1tsp) fresh coriander
5ml (1tsp) fresh parsley
5ml (1tsp) tomato purée
900ml (11/2 pints) vegetable stock or water seasoning
Optional: *Juice of 225g (1/2lb) carrots*

Sauté the onions and garlic in the olive oil until soft. Chop the carrots and add, along with the rest of the ingredients. Bring to the boil, add seasoning and leave to simmer for one hour. Add the carrot juice and liquidise. Can be served hot or cold with a little chopped parsley or coriander on top.

Root soup

    225g (¹/₂lb) onion
    225g (¹/₂lb) beetroot
    100g (4oz) parsnips
    100g (4oz) carrots
    100g (4oz) swede or turnip
    100g (4oz) potato
    5ml (1tsp) chopped parsley
    22.5ml (1¹/₂tbsp) yoghurt
    30ml (2tbsp) olive oil
    600ml (1 pint) vegetable stock/water seasoning
    Optional: Juice of 100g (4oz) parsnip and 100g (4oz) carrots

Chop the onions and sauté in the olive oil until tender. Chop the rest of the vegetables and add to the onions. Pour in the stock/water, bring to the boil, add parsley and seasoning, and leave to simmer for one hour. Add the vegetable juice and liquidise. Stir in the yoghurt before serving.

Tomato and orange soup

    750g (1¹/₂lbs) tomatoes
    225g (¹/₂lb) onions
    2 cloves garlic
    100g (4oz) carrots
    Juice of ¹/₂ orange, with a strip of the rind
    20ml (4tsp) tomato purée
    5ml (1tsp) mixed herbs
    1 bay leaf
    Seasoning

30ml (2tbsp) olive oil
600ml (1 pint) vegetable stock/water
Optional: *Juice of 6 tomatoes and 50g (2oz) onion*

Chop the onions and garlic and sauté in the oil until tender. Chop the tomatoes and carrots and add the onions and garlic. Add the orange juice and a strip of the rind, add the rest of the ingredients, season and bring to the boil. Simmer for about an hour. Remove the orange rind and the bay leaf, add the vegetable juice and liquidise. Serve hot.

Spicy mixed pepper soup

750g (1¹/₂lbs) different coloured peppers (red, yellow, green, orange)
¹/₂ chilli pepper
225g (¹/₂lb) onion
2 cloves garlic
100g (4oz) potatoes
225g (¹/₂lb) tomatoes
5ml (1tsp) tomato purée
5ml (1tsp) mixed herbs
5ml (1tsp) chopped parsley
30ml (2tbsp) olive oil
600ml (1 pint) vegetable stock/water
Seasoning
Parmesan cheese
Optional: *Juice of 6 tomatoes and 1 pepper*

Chop the onions, garlic and chilli pepper and sauté in the olive oil until tender. Chop the tomatoes and potato, slice the peppers and add to the pot. Add the rest of the ingredients (apart from the parmesan), bring to the boil, season and allow to simmer for about an hour. Add the vegetable juice and liquidise. Serve hot with a sprinkling of parmesan cheese on top.

—8—
Healthy Eating Plan

If you are unable to fast, you can still follow a new regime of healthier eating which will both encourage weight loss and better health. The World Health Organisation recommends we should eat about one pound of fruit and vegetables every day (excluding potatoes) if we want to keep fit and healthy. This means about five portions, but the average British diet includes only about half that amount. The Greeks and Spanish eat at least twice the amount of vegetables as us and this higher vegetable consumption is part of the 'Mediterranean diet effect' hailed as being responsible for lower rates of cancer and heart disease in Mediterranean countries. So the message is: if you want better health, go for at least five portions of fruit and vegetables every day.

By including fresh fruit and vegetable juices in your daily diet you can easily consume 1lb of fruit or vegetables. They can become part of your everyday diet and, if you are also aiming to lose weight, juices can help to curb your appetite and stimulate your metabolism.

A combined eating plan of juice and meals will still stimulate the body to eliminate toxins and repair damaged cells as long as meals are light and nutritious. (American 'Juiceman' Jay Korvich eats nearly all of his food raw – about 90 percent of his daily intake – and avoids meat, dairy products, sugar and coffee.) Just one or two juices a day will help to reap the benefits of better health. The combination of juice and food also ensures that we get adequate fibre in our diet. Studies worldwide show that fibre is a key component in preventing colon cancer. Fibre is essential for good bowel movement and for sweeping toxins out of the bowl like a broom. This is why health experts suggest we eat 'around a juicer' by eating plenty of high fibre foods like fruit and vegetables, whole grains and legumes, as well as drinking juices.

DAILY JUICING ALONG WITH HEALTHIER EATING ...
* flushes out toxins
* provides fluid to the cells
* replaces depleted vitamins and minerals
* builds up stores of nutrients for later use
* assists with regular bowel and urine production.

Ideally juices should be drunk half an hour before meals otherwise the sugars and starches in the juice can begin to ferment in the digestive tract while other food is still being digested and this can lead to all sorts of digestive upsets.

One-Week Healthy Eating Plan

INCLUDE:
* One to three fresh juices per day.
* One to two litres of filtered or bottled water.

BREAKFAST IDEAS
Fresh fruit
Fruit salad
Stewed fruit
Dried fruit compote
Prunes
Porridge with raisins or stewed apple
Herb teas
Hot water with lemon and ginger

LUNCH IDEAS

Raw vegetable salad with olive oil and lemon juice dressing
Baked or steamed potatoes
Brown rice, wild rice, brown Basmati rice
Sprouted seeds and beans
Vegetable soup
Avocado
Cottage cheese
Fruit

SUPPER IDEAS

Fresh fish – grilled or baked
Rice cakes and tahini (sesame paste)
Sweet potato – steamed
Baked potato
Vegetable stew with lentils or beans
Brown rice or millet
Lightly cooked vegetables – steamed
Stir-fried vegetables in olive oil
Salad with olive oil dressing
Fruit

SNACKS

Rice cakes
Vegetable crudities
Pumpkin seeds, sunflower seeds, sesame seeds, etc.
Banana

DRINKS

Fresh fruit or vegetable juices
Herb tea – camomile, dandelion, fennel, peppermint, etc.
Bottled or filtered water

Foods to avoid

  Meat
  Dairy produce – milk, cheese (only cottage cheese is allowed),
  butter, etc.
  Wheat – bread, pastry, cakes, biscuits
  Sauces
  Butter, margarine
  Eggs
  Sugar and salt
  Tea, coffee, alcohol
  Processed foods
  Fried food
  Saturated fats
  Chocolate
  Spicy foods

The above foods are a guide to what you can and can't eat on a one-week healthy eating plan which combines fresh fruit and vegetable juices with healthy meals. As with all roads to better health, exercise, correct breathing and a positive attitude are also important.

Almost everyone will benefit from incorporating fresh juice into their daily diet. It is easy to do too – have a juice instead of a cup of coffee or tea in the morning, or instead of a glass of wine in the evening. If you are at home during the day you could have a juice pick-me-up mid-morning or mid-afternoon. Once you start juicing it becomes a way of life that you won't want to give up.

A Juice For All Seasons

Spring tonic
> 2 apples
> 2 carrots
> 1/2 beetroot

Wash and slice the apples, wash and trim the carrots, peel the beetroot. Juice.

Summer cooler
> 3 carrots
> 1/4 cucumber
> 4 radishes

Wash and trim the carrots, wash and slice the cucumber. Juice.

Autumn daze
> 1 apple
> 1 pear
> 1/2lb black grapes (or blackberries)

Wash and slice the apple, wash and slice the pear, wash the grapes or blackberries. Juice.

Winter warmer
> 2 apples
> 1 orange
> 1cm cube of fresh ginger
> 2 carrots

Wash and slice the apples, peel the orange and ginger, trim the carrots. Juice.

Nutrient composition

For selected fruit and vegetables per 3¹/₂oz (100g) portion

Fruit or Vegetable	Bulk Nutrients			Minerals				
	P (g)	F (g)	C (g)	Ca (mg)	Mg (mg)	Na (mg)	K (mg)	Fe (mg)
Apple	0.2	0.6	14.5	7	6.4	1	110	0.3
Apricot	1.0	0.2	12.8	17	9.2	1	110	0.5
Asparagus	2.5	0.2	5	22	20	2	278	1.0
Beetroot	1.6	0.1	9.9	16	25	60	335	0.7
Blackberry	1.2	0.9	12.9	32	30	1	170	0.9
Broccoli	3.3	0.2	2	105	24	13	464	1.3
Cabbage	1.3	0.2	5.4	49	23	20	233	0.4
Carrot	1.1	0.2	9.7	37	18	47	341	0.3
Celery	0.9	0.1	3.9	39	12	126	341	0.3
Cranberry	0.4	0.7	7.8	14.4	7.2	1.8	90	0.9
Cucumber	0.6	0.2	2.2	15	8	8.5	141	0.5
Dandelion	2.6	0.6	–	158	36	76	440	3.1
Endive	1.7	0.1	4.1	81	10	14	294	1.7
Fennel	2.4	0.3	–	109	49	86	494	2.7
Grape	1.3	0.1	15.7	16	9.3	3	158	0.4
Grapefruit	0.5	0.1	10.6	16	10	1	135	0.4
Kale	6.0	8	9	249	37	75	378	2.7
Kiwi	1.0	0.6	10.3	38	23.8	4.1	295	0.8
Lemon	1.1	0.3	8.2	26	28	2	138	0.6
Lettuce	1.2	0.2	2.5	35	11	9	264	2
Lime	0.5	2.4	1.9	13	–	2	82	0.2
Mango	0.6	0.3	12.8	12	18	5	190	0.4
Melon (honeydew)	0.6	–	5	12	13	20	220	0.5
Orange	1.0	0.2	12.2	41	14	1	200	0.4
Papaya	0.6	0.1	10	20	40.5	3	234	0.3
Parsnip	1.7	0.5	17.5	50	22	12	541	0.7
Peach	0.6	0.1	9.7	9	9.2	1	202	0.5
Pear	0.7	0.4	15.3	8	7.8	2	130	0.3
Pepper (green)	1.2	0.2	4.8	9	–	13	213	0.7
Pineapple	0.4	0.2	13.7	17	17	1	146	0.5
Potato	2.1	0.1	17.1	7	25	3	407	0.6
Prunes	0.7	0.4	34	34	24	11	760	2.6
Radish	1.1	0.1	2.2	34	8	17	255	1.5
Raspberry	1.3	0.3	5.8	29	13	–	170	1
Spinach	3.2	0.3	4.3	93	58	71	470	3.1
Strawberry	0.7	0.5	8.4	21	15	1	164	1
Tomato	1.1	0.2	4.7	13	20	3	244	0.5
Turnip	1.0	0.2	6.6	39	7.4	49	268	0.5
Watercress	2.2	0.3	3.0	151	17	52	282	1.7
Watermelon	0.5	0.2	6.4	7	2.9	1	100	0.5

Abbreviations: P = protein, F = fat, C = carbohydrate, Ca = calcium, Mg = magnesium, Na = sodium, K = potassium, Fe = iron, Se = selenium, Io = Iodine, – = trace amounts only or none, g – grams, mg – milligrams, mcg – micrograms
Source: **Composition of Foods Handbook No 8.** *US Department of Agriculture.*

Se (mcg)	Io (mcg)	Beta-carotene (mg)	B3 (mg)	B5 (mg)	C (mg)	E (mg)	B1 (mcg)	B2 (mcg)	B6 (mcg)	Folic acid (mcg)
						VITAMINS				
0.9	–	0.05	0.3	0.1	12	0.49	35	32	45	6.5
–	0.5	1.79	0.77	0.29	9.4	0.5	40	53	70	3.6
–	7	0.03	1	0.62	21	2	110	120	60	86
0.8	–	0.01	0.23	–	10	0.03	22	42	50	93
–	–	0.27	0.4	0.22	17	0.72	30	40	50	–
–	–	0.9	0.23	–	10	0.03	22	42	50	93
18	5.2	0.04	0.32	0.26	45.8	1.7	48	43	110	79
–	–	12	0.58	0.27	7	0.6	69	53	93	8
–	–	0.02	0.55	0.43	7	–	48	76	90	7
–	–	0.02	0.1	–	18	–	30	20	–	30
–	2.5	0.17	0.2	0.24	8	0.1	18	30	35	20
–	–	7.9	0.8	–	30	2.5	190	170	–	–
3	6.4	1.14	0.41	–	9.4	–	52	120	–	49
–	–	4.7	0.2	0.25	93	–	23	110	100	100
2.8	0.7	0.03	0.23	0.06	4.2	–	46	25	73	5.4
0.2	1.3	0.02	0.24	0.25	44	0.25	48	24	28	11
2.3	12	4.1	2.1	–	105	1.7	100	250	250	60
–	–	0.37	0.41	–	71	–	17	50	–	–
1.2	0.5	0.02	0.07	0.27	53	–	17	50	–	–
0.8	3.3	0.8	0.32	0.11	13	0.44	62	78	55	37
–	–	0.01	0.17	–	43.5	–	28	20	–	–
–	1.6	2.8	0.7	–	38.7	1.0	45	50	–	36
–	–	0.1	0.5	0.23	25	0.1	50	30	70	30
3.5	2.1	0.09	0.3	0.24	50	0.24	79	42	50	24
–	–	0.56	0.3	–	24	–	30	39	–	–
–	3.6	0.2	0.94	0.5	18	1	80	130	110	–
0.4	1	0.44	0.85	0.14	9.5	–	27	51	26	2.7
1.2	1.5	0.03	0.22	0.06	4.6	0.43	33	38	15	14
–	2.3	0.2	0.33	0.23	139	3.1	60	50	270	17.5
–	–	0.06	0.22	0.18	19	0.1	72	43	75	4
–	3.8	0.01	1.22	0.4	17	0.06	110	47	210	7
3	–	0.14	1.3	0.41	–	–	90	180	210	3
–	8	0.02	0.25	0.18	29	–	33	30	60	24
–	–	0.08	0.3	0.3	25	0.48	23	50	75	–
1.7	12	4.2	0.62	0.25	52	1.6	110	230	220	78
–	1	0.05	0.51	0.3	64	0.12	31	54	60	16
0.6	1.7	0.82	0.53	0.31	24.2	0.82	57	35	100	39
–	7.5	0.06	0.67	0.2	20	–	40	51	80	20
–	–	3	0.6	0.1	60	1	85	100	130	–
–	1	0.2	0.15	1.6	6	–	45	50	70	5

Useful Addresses

British Register of Naturopathy
328 Harrogate Road, Moortown, Leeds LS17 6PE
Send an SAE for details of your nearest registered naturopath or details of training in naturopathy.

Gerson Institute
PO Box 430, Bonita, California 91908, USA
Tel: 00 1 (619) 267 1150
Cancer clinic and alternative treatment centre. Focus is on juice therapy.

Henry Doubleday Research Association
Bocking, Braintree, Essex CV8 3LG
Tel: 01203 303517
Largest organisation of organic gardeners in the world; new members are welcome. Products and gardening books available by mail order.

Wholistic Research Company
Bright Haven, Robin's Lane, Lolworth, Cambridge CB3 8HH
Tel: 01954 781074
Stockists of juicing equipment, water distillers and enema kits.

The Institute for Complementary Medicine
PO Box 194, London SE16 1QZ
Tel: 0171 237 5165
Contact the Institute for a list of practitioners in your area and details of courses in nutrition and naturopathy.

The Soil Association
86 Colston Street, Bristol BS1 5BB
Tel: 0117 9290661
Send an SAE for list of organic farmers and stockists in your area. The Soil Association symbol is a consumer guarantee that food is high quality and organically grown. New members are welcome.

World Cancer Research Fund
Freepost CV1037, Stratford-upon-Avon CV37 0BR
This charity studies the effects of diet on cancer. Send an SAE for a booklet entitled *ABC Guide to Reducing Your Cancer Risk*.

Index